ACTION PLAN FOR
ALLERGIES

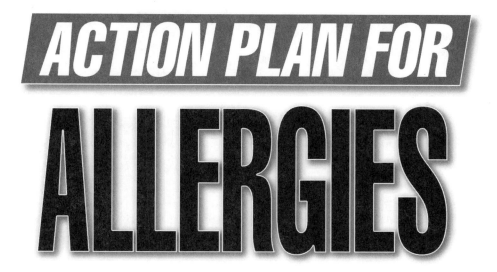

WILLIAM BRINER, MD

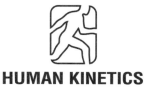

HUMAN KINETICS

Library of Congress Cataloging-in-Publication Data

Briner, William, 1958-
  Action plan for allergies / William Briner.
     p. cm.
  Includes bibliographical references and index.
  ISBN-13: 978-0-7360-6279-4 (soft cover)
  ISBN-10: 0-7360-6279-3 (soft cover)
  1. Allergy--Prevention. 2. Asthma--Prevention. 3. Allergy--Exercise therapy. 4.
Asthma--Exercise therapy. 5. Physical fitness. I. Title.
  RC584.B75 2007
  616.97'06--dc22

                       2006013909

ISBN-10: 0-7360-6279-3
ISBN-13: 978-0-7360-6279-4

The Web addresses cited in this text were current as of May 10, 2006, unless otherwise noted.

Acquisitions Editor: Martin Barnard; **Developmental Editor:** Leigh Keylock; **Assistant Editor:** Christine Horger; **Copyeditor:** Joanna Hatzopoulos; **Proofreader:** Erin Cler; **Indexer:** Betty Frizzéll; **Permission Manager:** Carly Breeding; **Graphic Designer:** Fred Starbird; **Graphic Artist:** Tara Welsch; **Photo Manager:** Laura Fitch; **Cover Designer:** Jack W. Davis; **Photographer (interior):** Kelly Huff, unless otherwise noted; **Art Manager:** Kareema McLendon-Foster; **Illustrator:** Kareema McLendon-Foster; **Printer:** United Graphics

ACSM Publication Committee Chair: Jeffrey L. Roitman, EdD, FACSM; **ACSM Communications and Public Information Committee Chair:** Harold W. Kohl, PhD, FACSM; **ACSM Group Publisher:** D. Mark Robertson; **ACSM Editorial Manager:** Lori A. Tish

We thank BodyTech in St. Joseph, Illinois, for assistance in providing the location for the photo shoot for this book.

Human Kinetics books are available at special discounts for bulk purchase. Special editions or book excerpts can also be created to specification. For details, contact the Special Sales Manager at Human Kinetics.

Printed in the United States of America   10   9   8   7   6   5   4   3   2   1

Human Kinetics
Web site: www.HumanKinetics.com

United States: Human Kinetics
P.O. Box 5076
Champaign, IL 61825-5076
800-747-4457
e-mail: humank@hkusa.com

Canada: Human Kinetics
475 Devonshire Road Unit 100
Windsor, ON N8Y 2L5
800-465-7301 (in Canada only)
e-mail: orders@hkcanada.com

Europe: Human Kinetics
107 Bradford Road
Stanningley
Leeds LS28 6AT, United Kingdom
+44 (0) 113 255 5665
e-mail: hk@hkeurope.com

Australia: Human Kinetics
57A Price Avenue
Lower Mitcham, South Australia 5062
08 8372 0999
e-mail: liaw@hkaustralia.com

New Zealand: Human Kinetics
Division of Sports Distributors NZ Ltd.
P.O. Box 300 226 Albany
North Shore City
Auckland
0064 9 448 1207
e-mail: info@humankinetics.co.nz

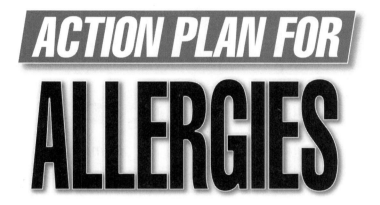

ACTION PLAN FOR ALLERGIES

CONTENTS

PREFACE

Almost everyone has allergies at one time or another. In fact, if we take the highest lifetime prevalence from published medical studies of the most common types of allergic symptoms, it becomes evident that allergic symptoms are practically universal. Studies show that up to 40 percent of people have symptomatic allergic rhinitis (hay fever) and 20 percent may have asthma, urticaria (hives), or atopic dermatitis (allergic rash). These figures do not even take into consideration several less common types of allergic disease. Some overlap exists between these conditions, so the same individual may be unfortunate enough to experience two or more of them, sometimes simultaneously. Unfortunately, recent studies also indicate that the frequency of respiratory allergies in particular is actually on the increase. Although exercise does not improve most allergy symptoms in and of itself, the question arises as to whether any reason exists for allergy patients to avoid exercise.

At a national sports medicine meeting, I presented a case of a patient with a condition called exercise-induced anaphylaxis, a severe, life-threatening allergic response to exercise. As I reviewed similar cases and discussed my case with experts, it became evident that most patients with this condition were actually regular exercisers. In fact, many were marathon runners. They adapted to their condition by injecting themselves with epinephrine (adrenaline) when they started to feel symptoms, and then they sometimes went on to complete the run. If these allergy patients can maintain an exercise program, then clearly anyone can. While some allergic conditions can be worsened by exercise in certain circumstances, no allergic disease qualifies as an excuse to avoid exercise. Exercise benefits everyone, and no allergic condition exists for which an exercise program to attain fitness and preventive medical goals is not reasonable. This book will give people with allergies the tools they need to use exercise to prevent disease and minimize their lifetime use of medication.

Most people are aware of the health benefits of exercise, but sometimes I wonder whether physicians have forgotten to adequately stress the importance of exercise to their patients. We expend huge amounts of effort and money to bring down bad cholesterol and high blood pressure *after* a heart attack, and we use an armamentarium of expensive new medications and injected insulin to tightly control blood sugar in people with diabetes. Insurance companies will pay for bariatric surgery to effectively bypass the stomach in markedly obese patients *and* their first plastic surgery to remove extra skin after they have lost thick layers of fat. Ample medical research demonstrates that all of these endeavors are reasonable in these populations, but they all fall into the category of secondary prevention. These people already have disease, and a predominant factor in all of these conditions is a sedentary lifestyle, or lack of exercise. Regular exercise can prevent some of these serious conditions and the expensive, invasive interventions that ensue. I am hopeful that this book will help those who suffer from allergies to realize that there are reasonable exercise options for them. Even if we view the issue from a cost/benefit perspective, it is clear that people with allergies who are able to maintain a regular exercise program will improve their health risk profile. They will be less likely to suffer adverse health care outcomes associated with a sedentary lifestyle, such as heart attack, stroke, or diabetes.

Allergy patients get the same benefits from exercise that everyone else does. For most allergic conditions, the concern is controlling symptoms to allow allergy sufferers to start and maintain an exercise program. For many conditions, some physical measures can even prevent symptoms from occurring. Certain types of exercise activity may be less likely to provoke symptoms while still allowing fitness goals to be achieved. Proper warm-up may also decrease the likelihood of allergic problems. Many of these conditions, though, require medications for adequate control. When medication is necessary, the recommendation in this book is for the minimal effective dose, and over-the-counter products are stressed when they are appropriate.

Allergies are ubiquitous, and literally hundreds of nonprescription preparations intended for their treatment are available. It is sometimes difficult to decide whether or not allergic symptoms need to be evaluated by a physician. Although it is not possible to give a definite answer to this question, this book provides general recommendations on when to seek medical care for each of the allergic conditions discussed.

Certainly most people with allergies are aware of their condition, but they may have associated symptoms that are also attributable to allergy. So, a chapter is devoted to recognizing symptoms and allergic triggers or allergens. The scientific basis of the allergic response also is reviewed. Then the components of fitness that are important to an exercise program are stressed. Aerobic (cardiovascular) fitness, strength, and flexibility are discussed with an emphasis on avoiding allergic symptoms during each of these activities. Some recommendations for varying activity to keep things interesting and tips on staying with a program are reviewed. Finally, individual allergic conditions are reviewed with special attention to exercise recommendations to decrease the likelihood of symptoms.

Regular exercisers are aware of the day-to-day benefits of a fitness program. In addition to decreasing the likelihood of illness and disability, most exercisers look forward to a sense of well-being during their exercise sessions. Those who adhere to a consistent aerobic program are less likely to experience symptoms of depression. As we will see in later chapters, people with allergies who do regular cardiovascular exercise often develop tolerance to the conditions that result in their allergic symptoms. Thus, they become able to enjoy a higher level of activity without symptoms. They may even be able to decrease the amount or frequency of medicines that they need to take. Read on for more information on how exercise can improve life for those with allergies and asthma.

William Briner, MD

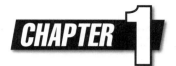

CHAPTER 1

TAKING CONTROL OF YOUR ALLERGIES

William Briner

Allergies are not a reason to avoid exercise. Athletes with asthma have competed at the highest levels of sport. For example, Jackie Joyner-Kersee won the gold medal twice in the Olympic heptathlon—a combination of events considered to determine the world's greatest female athlete—despite her asthma. Runners with exercise-induced anaphylaxis, a life-threatening allergic condition, have successfully completed marathons. For any given allergic condition, it is almost certain that a regimen of medical management and exercise training will allow those with asthma to engage in any activity level they desire. In fact, for allergic conditions that may be precipitated by exercise, it probably makes more sense to maintain a regular program of physical activity. It allows for desensitization to the allergic symptoms and should enable greater tolerance of exercise without provoking symptoms as activity is increased. The body's immune system mediates all allergy types. To understand allergies and their management, it is necessary to have a basic understanding of hypersensitivity and the immune system.

Hypersensitivity and the Immune System

The immune system is the body's mechanism for identifying and eliminating foreign substances and organisms that may be harmful to it. Allergic reactions are considered hypersensitivity reactions of the immune system. Hypersensitivity is a complex process of which several types exist. It will be considered only in a simplified form here. Most of the allergic reactions described in this book are immediate hypersensitivity reactions (also called type I hypersensitivity). A particle of pollen, a bacterium, or a virus is an allergen (antigen). Antibodies are present in the immune system to combine with allergens and eliminate them as a threat to the body. Immunoglobulin E (IgE) is the antibody involved in immediate hypersensitivity. The antigen-antibody complex (also called immune complex) causes the release of substances that cause blood vessels to increase in diameter (dilate) and the increased secretion from mucous glands, resulting in allergic symptoms. Histamine is one of the substances released from cells, which is why antihistamines may be an effective treatment for allergy symptoms. Leukotrienes are another substance released in hypersensitivity reactions. Physicians may prescribe medications that inhibit leukotrienes, such as montelukast (Singulair).

These events occur in almost all hypersensitivity reactions and are the reason people have common types of allergic symptoms. Fortunately, exercisers who understand their symptoms (and the factors that trigger them) can effectively prevent common allergic symptoms and exercise without being stifled by their allergies.

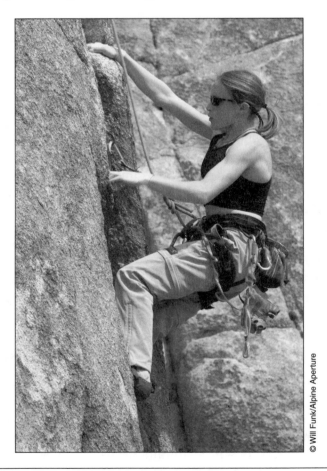

© Will Funk/Alpine Aperture

Allergies and asthma don't have to be activity-stoppers. Knowing your symptom triggers and planning ahead can help you head off barriers to staying active.

Asthma

Asthma may affect up to 5 percent of the population in the United States. It is most common in children. Some people "grow out of" their asthma, but it may occur at any age. Severe asthma attacks can be fatal, so asthma should be accurately diagnosed and optimally treated by a physician. Asthma is essentially an allergic condition of the lungs. The airways of people with asthma are sensitive to small particles in the air that they may be allergic to (such as pollen). These particles are called allergens. They may also be sensitive to irritants in the air such as sulfur dioxide, a component of air pollution. Exposure to these particles may result in swelling of the airway walls because of inflammation. The smooth muscle in the walls of the airways then goes into spasm, and more mucus is secreted into the airways. Narrowing of the airways results, and it precipitates an asthma attack.

The symptoms of an asthma attack may include wheezing, which is essentially noisy breathing because of the decreased diameter of the airway. Cough may occur. This cough may or may not be productive of phlegm or sputum. The individual may also experience shortness of breath, or "air hunger."

Exercise may cause an asthma attack in people who do not have the condition under control. It is particularly important to control airway inflammation. Prescription medications such as corticosteroids and leukotriene inhibitors may be needed. In some cases, other medications may be useful for long-term control of wheezing. Table 1.1 provides a list of these medications. A family doctor, pediatrician, internist, or pulmonologist (lung specialist) should manage asthma medications. Patients should meet with their physicians frequently until symptoms are under control. Patients who have been prescribed anti-inflammatory medications for their asthma almost always need to take them daily. Quick-relief, or "rescue," medicines, such as an albuterol inhaler, should be used infrequently. An albuterol inhaler should not be needed more than four times a week to control asthma symptoms. If it is used that often, a physician should recommend a different combination of medicines for better control of symptoms. (It is acceptable to use albuterol as often as daily to prevent exercise-induced asthma, as long as it is effective in keeping symptoms from occurring.) Usually, the best approach is for people with inflammatory asthma to become experts at recognizing their own symptoms, assessing the severity of asthma attacks, and managing prescribed medications accordingly. People who check their own peak flow at home are often best able to control their symptoms. The asthma action plan on page 7 can be used for recording this information. Keeping track of these details and reacting to them accordingly may help avoid severe, even fatal, asthma attacks. Once this baseline asthma has been controlled, it is usually safe to begin an exercise program.

Table 1.1 Asthma Medications

Anti-inflammatory medications		
Type of medicine	**Generic name**	**Brand name**
Corticosteroids, inhaled Potent anti-inflammatory	beclomethasone	Beclovent QVAR Vanceril Vanceril double strength
	budesonide	Pulmicort
	flunisolide	AeroBid AeroBid-M
	fluticasone	Flovent
	triamcinolone	Azmacort
Mast cell stabilizers, inhaled Anti-inflammatory or may be used before exposure to known trigger	cromolyn sodium nedocromil sodium	Intal Tilade
Other long-term control medications		
Type of medicine	**Generic name**	**Brand name**
Combined medication, inhaled Bronchodilator	ipratropium bromide + albuterol fluticasone + salmeterol	Combivent Advair
Long-acting beta2-agonists, inhaled or oral Bronchodilators	albuterol sulfate	Volmax Proventil Repetabs (tablet) VoSpire ER
	formoterol	Foradil
	salmeterol	Serevent

Type of medicine	Generic name	Brand name
Methylxanthine, oral bronchodilators Relax and open airways; stimulate diaphragm and breathing	theophylline	Aerolate III Aerolate JR Aerolate SR Choledyl SA Elixophyllin Quibron-T Quibron-T/SR Slo-bid Slo-Phyllin Theo-24 Theochron Theo-Dur Theolair Theolair SR T-Phyl Uni-Dur Uniphyl

Quick-relief medicines		
Type of medicine	**Generic name**	**Brand name**
Short-acting beta2-agonists, inhaled or oral Bronchodilators	albuterol	Airet Accuneb Proventil Proventil HFA Ventolin Ventolin Rotacaps Ventolin HFA
	bitoiterol	Tornalate
	pirbuterol	Maxair
	terbutaline	Brethaire
	levalbuterol	Brethine (tabs only) Bricanyl (tabs only) Xopenex

(continued)

Table 1.1   *(continued)*

Quick-relief medicines		
Type of medicine	**Generic name**	**Brand name**
Anticholinergics, inhaled Bronchodilator	ipratropium bromide	Atrovent
Additional medicines		
Type of medicine	**Generic name**	**Brand name**
Corticosteroids, oral Most potent anti-inflammatory May be used for short-term management or in long-term control	dexamethasone	Decadron Deltasone
	prednisolone	Pediapred Prelone Hydrocortone Medrol
	hydrocortisone	Prednisone
	methylprednisolone	Deltasone
	prednisone	Orasone Liquid Pred Prednisone Intensol

Exercise-Induced Asthma

Exercise-induced asthma (EIA) is a common condition that may affect 10 to 15 percent of the U.S. population. So, it is much more common than asthma itself. It probably occurs in susceptible individuals because their airways have an allergic reaction to the large volumes of cool, dry air inhaled during exercise. People can almost always prevent this response by taking two puffs of a beta-agonist bronchodilator medicine, such as albuterol, 15 minutes before exercise. For any individual with asthmatic symptoms related to exercise, medication is far more effective if taken before exercise. Symptoms may be much more severe and necessitate stopping exercise if the wheezing or cough occurs before taking the medication.

For patients with asthma that is not properly controlled, exercise will produce an asthma attack. The two components to asthma, inflammation and bronchospasm, are both results of an allergic reaction in the lungs. Inflammation was discussed earlier. Left uncontrolled, inflammation may lead to severe, even fatal attacks. Bronchospasm, thought to be the primary process occurring in EIA, results in tightening of the smooth muscle in the bronchioles (small airways) in the lungs. Usually an inhaler such

Asthma Action Plan

Asthma Action Plan for _____ Date _____

Doctor's name _____

Doctor's phone number _____

Hospital/emergency room phone number _____

GREEN ZONE: DOING WELL

▸ Experience no coughing, wheezing, chest tightness, or shortness of breath during the day or night, and

▸ Can do usual activities

And, if a peak flow meter is used:

Peak flow: more than _____
(80 percent or more of my best peak flow)

My best peak flow: _____

Take these long-term-control medicines each day (include an anti-inflammatory):

Medicine	How much to take	When to take it

YELLOW ZONE: ASTHMA IS GETTING WORSE

▸ Experience coughing, wheezing, chest tightness, or shortness of breath, or

▸ Experience night waking because of asthma, or

▸ Can do some but not all usual activities

Or

Peak flow: _____ to _____ (50-80 percent of my best peak flow)

First, add the following quick-relief medicine, and keep taking your Green Zone medicine: _____ (short-acting beta2-agonist)

Please circle one of the following:

▸ Two puffs every 20 minutes for up to 1 hour

▸ Four puffs every 20 minutes for up to 1 hour

▸ Nebulizer once

From *Action Plan for Allergies* by William Briner, 2007, Champaign, IL: Human Kinetics.

(continued)

(continued)

Second, if your symptoms (and peak flow, if used) return to Green Zone after 1 hour of above treatment:

(Please circle one or both of the following)

▸ Take the quick-relief medicine every 4 hours for 1 to 2 days.

▸ Double the dose of your inhaled steroid for _____ (7-10) days.

Or

If your symptoms (and peak flow, if used) do not return to Green Zone after 1 hour of above treatment:

(Please circle one, two, or all of the following)

▸ Take (short-acting beta-agonist) _____ two or four puffs or nebulizer.

▸ Add (oral steroid) _____ mg a day, for _____ (3-10) days.

▸ Call the doctor within _____ hours after taking the oral steroid.

RED ZONE: MEDICAL ALERT!

▸ Very short of breath, or

▸ Quick-relief medicines have not helped, or

▸ Cannot do usual activities, or

▸ Symptoms are same or get worse after 24 hours in the Yellow Zone

Or

Peak flow: less than _____ (50 percent of my best peak flow)

Take this medicine: _____ (short-acting beta-agonist)

Please circle one of the following:

▸ Four puffs

▸ Six puffs

▸ Nebulizer

Or

_____mg (oral steroid)

Then call your family doctor NOW.

Go to the hospital or call for an ambulance if you are still in the Red Zone after 15 minutes and you have not reached your doctor.

DANGER SIGNS

▸ Have trouble walking and talking from shortness of breath

▸ Lips or fingernails are blue

Take four or six puffs (please circle) of your quick-relief medicine and go to the hospital or call an ambulance (phone number _____) NOW!

From *Action Plan for Allergies* by William Briner, 2007, Champaign, IL: Human Kinetics.

Reprinted with permission, © 2006 American Lung Association

For more information about the American Lung Association or to support the work it does, call 1-800-LUNG-USA (1-800-586-4872) or log on to www.lungusa.org.

as albuterol can help control bronchospasm. Inflammation and broncho-spasm combine to cause airway narrowing, which results in wheezing and shortness of breath. Some affected individuals experience coughing with an asthma attack.

People who suspect they may have EIA should see a physician and be tested for it. EIA occurs far more frequently than it is diagnosed. Athletes who become short of breath more easily than teammates during the same activity and those who cough after exercise should be tested. EIA is more likely to occur with sustained strenuous activity lasting 3 to 5 minutes, so it is less often seen in sports such as baseball that involve short sprints. Long-distance runners who run for 10 minutes or longer also seem to be less likely to experience symptoms. Middle-distance runners, soccer play-ers, and basketball players are more likely to be affected.

Because EIA occurs secondary to cooling and drying of the airways when large volumes of air are inspired with exercise, activities performed in cool, dry air, such as ice skating, are likely to cause an attack. Swimming is reported to be the safest sport, probably because swimmers breathe warm, humid air.

Evaluation

If you think you may have EIA, it is reasonable to get the condition di-agnosed and treated. Some physicians will elect to simply treat patients with symptoms that sound like EIA, but other conditions that may cause similar symptoms do exist. Therefore, it is best to be evaluated for EIA. Treatment is usually easy, and athletes almost always say their perfor-mance is improved after treatment.

Most primary care sports medicine physicians are comfortable doing EIA testing. A good test should involve a measurement of lung function before and after exercise. The physician may measure lung volumes (spirometry) or simply how fast air can be expired (peak flow). Both are measures of the obstruction that occurs because of airway narrowing with asthma. More important than the respiratory evaluation is the intensity of the exercise. A sustained effort for at least 8 minutes at as high an intensity as possible will yield the most accurate results. Usually physicians have their patients use a treadmill or stationary bicycle, but the most practi-cal test is the one in which they measure lung function before and after the activity that causes symptoms. Sometimes it is necessary to bring a spirometer or peak flow meter to the practice facility.

Treatment

Almost all patients respond favorably to a prescription metered dose in-haler. Take these medicines as your doctor recommends them. In EIA, they are only effective if taken before exercise. Once you have been diagnosed with EIA, it is important to keep your inhaler with you and use it before exercise. Two of the beta-agonist medicines that are used in this way are albuterol and salmeterol. Albuterol lasts for 4 to 5 hours and should be taken as two puffs 15 minutes before exercise. Salmeterol lasts up to 9 hours and should be dosed 1 hour before starting exercise. Some athletes elect to simply use it twice daily. For individuals with baseline asthma, taking their beta-agonist in this fashion will work to control the bronchospasm of their EIA, if their inflammatory asthma is under control.

Proper inhaler technique is essential for successful EIA management. The easiest way to ensure proper technique is to use a spacer. A spacer is a device about the size of a soda can that enables inhalation of the aerosolized medicine into the small airways of the lung (see figure 1.1). Place the lips on the spacer and squeeze the inhaler, emitting a puff of medicine. Then, inhale as deeply as possible. If you don't use a spacer, remember not to place the lips directly on the inhaler because most of the medicine will get stuck on the moist mucous membranes of the inside of the mouth. Rather, place the inhaler about an inch outside the open mouth, then breathe in deeply, just after depressing the inhaler (see figure 1.2).

Hay Fever

Hay fever, allergic rhinitis (runny nose), and atopy are all essentially names for the same thing. Allergic rhinitis affects up to 25 percent of the U.S. population. Clear drainage from the nose; red, watery eyes; and sneezing all occur with exposure to allergens in the environment. Pollens and pol-

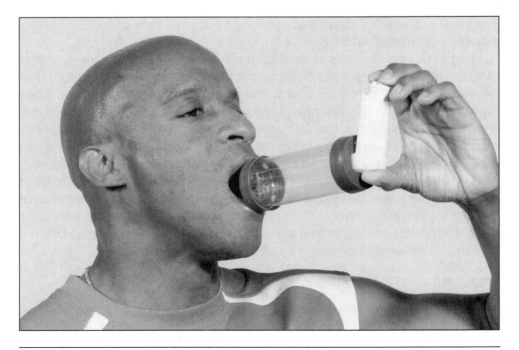

Figure 1.1 Proper use of a spacer.

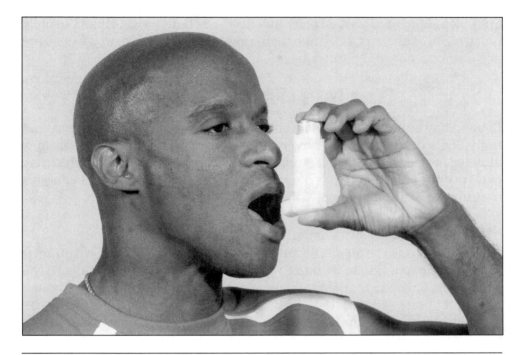

Figure 1.2   Proper use of an inhaler.

lutants in the air may be outdoor triggers. Dust and mold may be indoor triggers for susceptible individuals. Those who know that they are allergic to pollens should avoid outdoor exercise between the hours of 4 a.m. and 10 a.m. when pollen is airborne.

Unlike with asthma, exercise itself is not likely to cause hay fever symptoms. However, during exercise we inspire 100 times the volume of air than when at rest, so if a triggering allergen is present in the environment, it is more likely to produce symptoms with exercise. Fortunately, over-the-counter antihistamines can effectively prevent most symptoms.

Loratadine (e.g., Claritin) taken once daily will often alleviate allergic symptoms and allow an individual to return to exercise. This medication falls into the category of nonsedating antihistamines. These medications may be taken as needed to control symptoms during seasons when symptoms occur. Nonsedating antihistamines rarely result in problematic side effects.

Some individuals have perennial allergic rhinitis, with hay fever–type symptoms occurring throughout the year. These exercisers may wish to consider a sedating antihistamine such as diphenhydramine (e.g., Benadryl), especially if they experience symptoms on a daily basis. This medication is often useful for controlling symptoms, and the sedating antihistamines as a group are less expensive. The most common side effect is drowsiness, followed by dry mouth. However, if these medicines are taken daily for 2 weeks, tolerance to the sedative side effects usually occurs. So, exercisers who take them regularly for more than 2 weeks are not often bothered by drowsiness.

Other Types of Allergic Symptoms

EIA and hay fever are the most common allergic conditions that may affect individuals during exercise. Several other types of allergic symptoms may afflict exercisers, too. In fact, some rare allergic conditions exist that may even occur as a direct result of exercise. Other types of physical allergies may also affect active people.

Hives

Hives (urticaria) are also referred to as the "wheal and flare" reaction. It is an allergic reaction in the superficial dermis, which is just beneath the epidermis, or top layer of skin. This results in a raised itchy area, about a half-inch in size (wheal). Usually redness (flare) surrounds it. The cause of most hives is not known, often even in patients who have had extensive testing to try to determine the allergic trigger that initiates hives. For this reason, it may be more reasonable to simply treat the condition rather than subject the patient to exhaustive evaluation. When a cause is identified, drugs, foods, insect bites, and viral infections are the most common inciting allergens.

Antihistamines (particularly diphenhydramine and hydroxyzine) are often helpful in controlling hives. In rare situations, hives may occur with physical activity (see Physical Allergies).

Angioedema

Angioedema is essentially the same process as urticaria except that it occurs in the deeper layer of the dermis. Therefore, swelling is the main manifestation, and this swelling can be painful. You can see it on the hands, feet, face, and mouth (pharynx). The most severe form of angioedema involves the throat. Swelling can squeeze off the airway, even resulting in death. The treatment for this sort of angioedema is urgent injection of epinephrine, usually by a physician in the emergency room (see the next section on anaphylaxis). A specific cause is identified more often for angioedema than for hives, possibly because it is more likely to be a life-threatening condition, so it may be necessary to search harder to identify a cause. Again, the common causes are drugs, foods, insect bites, and viral infections.

Anaphylaxis

Anaphylaxis is a severe, life-threatening allergic reaction. Hives, angioedema, and very low blood pressure may all occur quickly. Angioedema must always be treated by an epinephrine injection. Although it is a serious condition, individuals who have had episodes of anaphylaxis can still exercise. If you have this condition, you should see a physician and get a prescription for an epinephrine preparation that can be self-injected (e.g., EpiPen, Ana-Kit) and keep it with you when you exercise. Because anaphylaxis is a potentially fatal condition, a search for its cause is probably worth pursuing for most every patient. The most common causes are foods and insect stings.

Insect Sting Allergy

The painful sensation that everyone feels when stung by a bee is, in fact, an immediate hypersensitivity allergic reaction. Most people experience a local reaction with swelling and redness up to 2 inches in diameter. Some people may have a more extensive local reaction with swelling of an entire limb. Such a reaction can usually be treated with a painkilling spray, an antihistamine gel applied to the area, or an antihistamine taken by mouth. A much more serious reaction is a generalized allergic reaction to an insect sting. Anaphylaxis or angioedema involving the airway must be taken very seriously. Patients with a history of severe allergic reaction to insect stings should, at minimum, be prescribed epinephrine (e.g., EpiPen, Ana-Kit) to self-administer if they are stung again.

About 50 percent of people will have a severe reaction to a bee sting after they have had one such reaction. So, another treatment option to consider is desensitization shots by an allergist (see chapter 6). This treatment may be particularly appropriate in individuals who continue exercising out of doors during summer months after the diagnosis has been made. After this series of shots, the individual will no longer have generalized symptoms after a bee sting if the treatment is successful.

Physical Allergies

Physical allergies are a group of allergic conditions that may occur either directly because of exercise or secondary to physical conditions that may be present in the exercise environment.

Exercise-Induced Anaphylaxis

Patients who have this rare condition have the most severe type of allergic reaction to exercise itself. In anaphylaxis, angioedema may occur, resulting in swelling of the throat and blockage of the upper airway. Mediator substances may be released into the blood, possibly resulting in a severe decrease in blood pressure (vascular collapse) because of dilation (opening up) of the blood vessels. Also, large hives develop.

Symptoms occur intermittently with exercise. An attack is usually preceded by itchy skin and sometimes by a feeling of light-headedness that occurs during exercise. Then the hives typically occur, followed by angioedema or vascular collapse. Unfortunately, no medication has been effective in preventing attacks. Individuals with exercise-induced ana- phylaxis (EIAx) should be prescribed an EpiPen by a physician, and they should feel comfortable with its use. This device allows the individual to rapidly inject epinephrine under the skin, which is usually effective in halt- ing an attack. They should be advised to always exercise with a partner who understands their condition and can also administer epinephrine.

EIAx patients may need to alter their exercise regimen to avoid activi- ties known to cause symptoms. Anaphylaxis is more likely to occur after eating, so exercising 4 or more hours after the last meal may decrease the likelihood of attacks. Up to 30 percent of EIAx patients' symptoms are triggered by a specific food. Skin testing by an allergist should be under- taken to attempt to identify such foods. Then these foods can be avoided, particularly prior to exercise. Women may be more likely to have attacks around the time of their period. Anti-inflammatory medicines, such as ibuprofen, seem also to increase the risk of attack, so EIAx patients should avoid them. Although patients with this condition face a high risk of severe illness and even death with exercise, most are able to manage their condi- tion and plan their exercise so that they are able to remain active.

Cholinergic Urticaria

Cholinergic urticaria (CU) causes very small hives to occur with exercise, stress, or passive warming, such as might occur in a hot tub. Any situation that results in a 2-degree increase in temperature will cause these itchy hives to occur in afflicted individuals. In most people with CU, symptoms occur every time this happens. Wheezing similar to that which is seen in asthma may occur. Fortunately, this is a condition that can almost al- ways be successfully treated. The most effective medicine is hydroxyzine (e.g., Atarax). It is an antihistamine with anticholinergic effects that are probably beneficial in treatment. Hydroxyzine is a sedating antihistamine that may cause drowsiness with the first few doses. CU patients should take daily the lowest dose of hydroxyzine that is effective in preventing symptoms. The drowsiness almost always resolves within 2 weeks. With CU, hydroxyzine usually needs to be taken long term.

Cold Urticaria

In this condition, hives occur on the skin with exposure to cold. It may be particularly problematic in swimmers, ice skaters, and other winter sport participants. The condition may be diagnosed with an ice cube test, in which an ice cube is placed on the skin of the forearm for 4 minutes. A hive will occur in this spot in afflicted individuals. It can usually be treated successfully with cyproheptadine (Periactin), an antihistamine. Again, pa- tients should take the lowest effective dose on a daily basis to decrease the likelihood of drowsiness. Again, long-term treatment is usually needed.

Solar Urticaria

In this condition, very small wheals occur intermittently with sun exposure. Patients with solar urticaria should avoid medications that may increase sensitivity to the sun's rays (e.g., tetracycline, erythromycin, and other antibiotics). Individuals who have experienced this condition, which is sometimes referred to as "sun poisoning," should always apply a sunscreen with an SPF of at least 30 to exposed skin when sun exposure is unavoidable. Keeping the skin covered with a long-sleeved shirt and long pants also prevents solar urticaria.

Taking Control

Everyone with allergies can find an exercise regimen that will allow them to work toward their fitness goals. For most people, it involves taking the appropriate medication before potential allergic exposures. For some, adjustments in exercise routine will allow them to become more tolerant of their allergies. They may become desensitized to their allergic conditions as they increase their exercise intensity and duration. This and other important issues for patients with allergies will be addressed in future chapters.

Many of the aspects of an exercise prescription for allergy patients are not significantly different from those for the general population. Certainly, individuals with allergies derive all of the same physiologic benefits of exercise that everyone else does. The specifics of designing an exercise program for allergy patients are discussed in chapter 2. Aerobic activity, strength, and flexibility are addressed in later chapters. All of the information an allergy sufferer needs to initiate or fine-tune an exercise program is presented in a straightforward fashion.

Summary

Asthma and hay fever are the two most common types of allergic conditions that affect exercisers. Before starting an exercise program, the patient must work with a physician to control inflammation of baseline asthma using prescription medication. Exercise-induced asthma should be diagnosed with an exercise challenge test. Usually it can be treated with a beta-agonist inhaler such as albuterol before exercise. Hay fever can often be controlled with over-the-counter antihistamines that will allow symptom-free exercise.

Angioedema, hives, and anaphylaxis are potentially serious allergic conditions that must be evaluated and treated by a physician before an exercise program is initiated. Exercise-induced anaphylaxis is a very rare condition in which exercise itself may cause a life-threatening allergic reaction. However, many people who have this condition have been able to continue exercising if they keep epinephrine for self-administration handy. Hives may also occur in cholinergic urticaria when a person exercises or is psychologically stressed. It can be treated with prescription hydroxyzine. Cold urticaria (or hives) is treated with cyproheptadine by prescription. Note that hydroxyzine and cyproheptadine may cause drowsiness, but patients usually develop a tolerance to this side effect after taking these medications consistently over 2 weeks. These medicines are also more effective in treating these conditions when taken every day. Solar hives may be effectively managed in active patients with a combination of sun exposure avoidance and sunscreen use.

People who have allergies need not think of their condition as an impediment to exercise. The management schemes described in this chapter should allow most allergy patients to get started with an exercise program. Depending on your fitness goals, you may be able to increase the duration and intensity of your exercise sessions. The following chapters address the important components of fitness for exercisers with allergies. They also address some nonmedical approaches to allergy management.

ACTION PLAN:
TAKING CONTROL OF YOUR ALLERGIES

- ☐ Think of allergies as a hurdle to cross in your exercise program, not as an excuse to avoid exercising.
- ☐ Be sure that baseline asthma is under control before starting an exercise program.
- ☐ If you are unsure whether you may have exercise-induced asthma, get evaluated by a physician.
- ☐ Use your albuterol inhaler before exercise to prevent exercise-induced asthma.
- ☐ Take antihistamines on a daily basis to control allergic rhinitis or hay fever.
- ☐ Follow your doctor's advice, and take your medication if you have been diagnosed with a physical allergy.

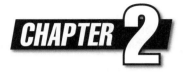

CHAPTER 2

DESIGNING AN EXERCISE PROGRAM

William Briner

People usually go through a progression of thought processes as they initiate a behavior pattern such as a new exercise program (Prochaska and DiClemente 1983). Most people go through a contemplative stage when considering starting an exercise program, and they may try to gain more information about various aspects of fitness (such as the information in this book). Next comes the planning phase, when they use this information to set forth fitness goals and incorporate them into an exercise regimen. Then comes the action stage, when they begin exercise activity. Adherence to an exercise program requires a long-term maintenance stage, during which they continue exercise behavior. You can use the information in this chapter to help you start the first stage of goal setting, but it is intended for allergy patients who have committed themselves to maintaining an exercise program. So be prepared to get to the final stage. This chapter provides a review of the components of an exercise prescription, including flexibility and strength training recommendations. It also discusses frequency, intensity, and duration of aerobic exercise to maximize weight loss or gain a cardiovascular training effect. Where appropriate, the chapter offers specific suggestions to minimize allergic symptoms during exercise.

Setting Goals

Carefully consider your fitness goals when starting an exercise program. Many people start exercising with a vague idea about losing weight, become frustrated when weight loss hasn't occurred after 3 weeks, and abandon their whole exercise plan. Consider realistic, attainable goals that you can assess and reassess. Attaining your goals can be a source of satisfaction that helps you maintain exercise behavior. Some examples of appropriate goals follow.

Short-Term Goals Short-term goals can be achieved over 2 weeks. Such a goal might be as simple as "Increase how long I can spend walking from 10 to 20 minutes without wheezing or coughing." You might achieve this goal by increasing walking time by 1 minute during each exercise session over 5 days each week. This gradual increase in exercise duration allows for tolerance to allergic symptoms to occur as the goal is attained. If you have symptoms that make exercise difficult on a particular day, you may need to modify your goals that day.

Long-Term Goals Long-term goals may be achieved over many months. It is probably best to consider weight loss as a long-term goal. A man who is 5 feet, 9 inches tall and weighs 245 pounds may set long-term goals of losing 5 pounds over 2 months and 15 pounds over 6 months. Allergic symptoms need to be controlled at the outset of a program that addresses long-term

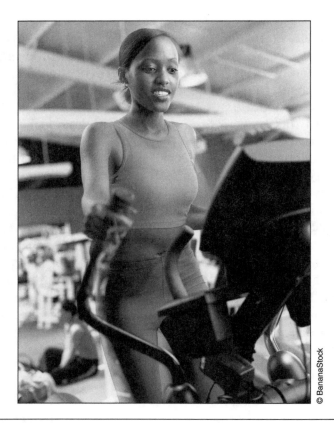

© BananaStock

Some of the most satisfying goals to reach will be ones that are specifically built around allergies and asthma—for example, setting a goal to gradually increase your exercise intensity without wheezing.

goals. In general, exercisers who need prescription or over-the-counter medicines to treat symptoms at the start of an exercise program should continue using those medications to get closer to their exercise goals.

Consulting a Physician About Exercise

Consult a physician before you start a new exercise program if you fit into any of these categories:

▸ Any aspect of your allergies is not under control.

▸ You are over the age of 35.

▸ You have two or more cardiac risk factors—smoking, high blood pressure, obesity (body mass index greater than 30), diabetes, high cholesterol (or if you don't know your cholesterol), or family history of heart disease.

▸ You have chest pain, shortness of breath, passing out, or dizziness with exercise.

Some reasonably fit adults who have exercised regularly without problems within the past few years can gradually initiate an exercise program (such as a walking program) without a physician's input. If you don't have any of the cardiac risk factors discussed, you have a body mass index less than 27 (see table 2.1 on page 24), and within the last 2 years you have been able to exercise at least three times weekly for at least 30 minutes at an intensity where you have worked up a sweat, you probably fall into this category.

Components of Fitness

An effective exercise program needs to address all of the components of fitness. You can improve endurance, or stamina, mostly with aerobic, or cardiovascular, exercise. Other essential elements in a fitness program are strength training, which usually requires resistance exercises, and flexibility, which you can improve through stretching.

Aerobic Exercise

Aerobic exercise (or cardiovascular fitness) is the most important component of a fitness program. Unfortunately, aerobic training is also the type of exercise that is most likely to provoke respiratory allergies.

Because the volume of inspired air may increase by 50 to 100 times that at baseline, whatever allergens are present in the environment that may provoke symptoms may be more likely to do so with exercise. Typically, premedication with an antihistamine or inhaler (see chapter 1) before strenuous aerobic exercise will help to alleviate symptoms.

Aerobic exercise uses the large muscles in the body (especially in the thighs) rhythmically over the course of time. This activity results in an increased heart rate and improved endurance for the heart muscle and the skeletal muscles involved. The American College of Sports Medicine (ACSM) recommends accumulating 30 minutes or more of moderate-intensity physical activity on most, and preferably all, days of the week. Any amount of aerobic activity can improve a person's functional capacity, but to achieve a cardiovascular training effect, a person must meet minimal parameters. This training effect allows for improvement in capacity for endurance exercise over the course of time. To attain a training effect, you must consider frequency, duration, and intensity. A minimal amount of aerobic exercise to achieve this effect is 20 minutes in duration, with a frequency of at least three times a week, at an intensity level at least where sweating occurs.

Frequency

As noted, a training effect requires a minimum frequency of three times a week. In general, improvement in cardiovascular fitness (and maintenance of fitness) occurs with increasing frequency of cardiovascular exercise up to 6 days a week. Allowing a day of rest from aerobic activity each week probably helps to prevent tissue breakdown and overuse injury.

Duration

Twenty minutes of continuous aerobic activity is needed for improving the endurance of the heart muscle. Lesser amounts of activity are certainly better than no exercise at all, but 20 minutes is the minimum duration for a training effect. Cardiovascular fitness continues to improve with increasing duration up to about 1 hour. Of course, a longer duration may be beneficial in training for certain types of competition such as marathon running.

If weight loss is your exercise goal, duration is the most important parameter of cardiovascular exercise. The body begins using fat tissue and free fatty acids as fuel for exercising after about 40 minutes of exercise. Before this point, it uses carbohydrate stored in the muscle and liver. Therefore, exercising for 1 hour, 6 days a week is probably the best program for weight loss. If time constraints preclude this amount of exercise, then alternating between 30 and 60 minutes of exercise over 6 days may be the next best option.

Intensity

Oxygen consumption, or $\dot{V}O_2$, is a measure of the amount of oxygen used by the body during exercise. The maximal $\dot{V}O_2$ is the amount of oxygen your lungs can take in during peak intensity of exercise ($\dot{V}O_2$max). For most exercisers, the ideal intensity with which to perform cardiovascular exercise is at 65 to 85 percent of their $\dot{V}O_2$max. Some people who have been sedentary for many years may gain cardiovascular benefit from training at 50 or even 40 percent of their $\dot{V}O_2$max. $\dot{V}O_2$max is essentially an all-out, 100 percent effort. Exercisers can assess exercise intensity in several ways. Most exercisers are achieving a training heart rate by working up a sweat. Research shows that exercisers are fairly accurate at gauging their own exercise intensity (Robertson et al. 2004).

Another method for determining exercise intensity is taking your pulse (see chapter 3). The most accurate equation for exercise intensity using resting heart rate (RHR) and your age is the Karvonen formula:

$$220 - \text{age} = X$$
$$X - RHR = Y$$
$$Y \text{ (65 to 85 percent of maximum heart rate)} = Z$$
$$Z + RHR = \text{training heart rate}$$

So, for a 47-year-old with a resting pulse of 60 who wants to train at 75 percent of maximum, the training heart rate would be

$$220 - 47 = 173$$
$$173 - 60 = 113$$
$$113 \ (.75) = 84.75$$
$$84.75 + 60 = 144.75.$$

People with exercise-induced asthma (EIA) may have a threshold phenomenon with respect to exercise intensity. It seems that exercise closer to maximum intensity lasting 4 to 8 minutes (such as a mile run) is more likely to promote symptoms than a longer duration of exercise at a lower intensity. So, exercising for 40 minutes on a stepper machine may be better tolerated than playing full-court basketball for 10 minutes. Or, put another way, it may be a better option for the exercise-induced asthma (EIA) patient to exercise at 65 percent of maximal heart rate rather than 85 percent.

Strength Training

Strength training is also referred to as weight training or resistance training. Improving strength is an important component of fitness and may enhance a person's functional ability to perform usual tasks of daily living. It may be particularly beneficial for older exercisers. For those who have respiratory allergy, resistance training is less likely to provoke symptoms than intensive cardiovascular exercise.

For most exercisers, the objective of resistance exercise is to increase muscle strength. Other benefits are increased lean body mass (relative to fat) and the body's improved ability to utilize nutrients (or burn calories). Periodization refers to the frequency of resistance exercise. To increase strength, you must strength train at least twice a week. You will have little increased benefit by working a muscle group more than four times a week. To avoid overuse injury and allow your muscles to recover, you should rest the muscles used for at least 1 day before training them again.

Other elements of periodization are the number of repetitions and sets of a given exercise needed for increasing strength. A repetition (rep) is one episode of an exercise, such as a biceps curl. A set is a given number of repetitions, such as a set of 12 reps of curls. No universal consensus on these recommendations exists, but for most exercisers, between 8 and 15 repetitions of an exercise is most likely beneficial. If maximal strength gains and muscle hypertrophy were the goal, then 8 repetitions would be optimal. Hypertrophy is the increase in muscle size that occurs as a result of resistance training. Individual muscle fibers cause this effect when they increase in diameter. If muscle endurance were the objective, then 12 to 15 repetitions would probably be more beneficial. In general, fewer repetitions with longer rest periods between sets are less likely to provoke respiratory allergy symptoms.

The correct amount of weight is the amount that can barely be raised and lowered under control with good form on the last repetition of the set. Performing 2 or 3 sets can lead to increased strength, whereas performing a single set is appropriate for maintaining strength.

Overload

The principle of overload states simply that when increased resistance is applied against exercising muscles, fitness gains occur. This principle operates with all forms of fitness activity, but it is most relevant for resistance exercise. Progressive resistance exercise means gradually increasing resistance from day to day and week to week. For example, you might add 10 pounds of resistance every 2 weeks when doing leg presses (2 sets of 10, 3 days per week) over the course of 6 months to increase your quadriceps strength.

The extent to which these principles are used in a fitness program will vary depending on your own fitness goals. Increases in weight may not be a necessary part of a program for strength maintenance.

Specificity

This principle states that the specific resistance exercise performed enhances the strength of the muscles used in that exercise. So, you must carefully choose resistance exercises that strengthen muscles specific to your long-term exercise activity. For instance, a volleyball player may choose 3 sets of 10 repetitions of leg presses and calf raises as part of a program to enhance strength in the muscles used for jumping.

Reversibility

Unfortunately, all of the fitness benefits that are gained via an exercise program can be lost fairly quickly. This is the principle of reversibility. Such losses can occur as quickly as just a few weeks. Reversibility can be an important motivator to maintain a fitness program over the course of time. Otherwise, strength and cardiovascular fitness and body composition return to their preexercise baseline.

Flexibility

Flexibility is the maintenance or enhancement of the body's range of motion, particularly in the arms and legs. You can use stretching exercises to enhance flexibility. The benefits of stretching are a bit difficult to discern from the sports medicine literature. Nonetheless, most exercise specialists recommend some stretching activity to maintain functional range of motion of the joints as part of an exercise program. It is particularly helpful if decreased range of motion or stiffness in a joint exists. These problems can occur with an injury such as a muscle pull or with arthritis.

Static stretching is holding a joint at the end of the range of motion for a count of time, then relaxing, then repeating the stretch five times. The modified hurdler's stretch is an example of a static stretch (see page 107). This sort of stretching may be helpful in restoring range of motion to a stiff joint or muscle. Ballistic stretching involves placing a muscle at the limit of its range of motion, then using a bouncing movement to stretch the muscle even farther. Stretch receptors in the muscle usually cause a reflex contraction during ballistic stretches. This action may increase the chance of injury during the stretch, so ballistic stretching is not generally recommended.

Dynamic stretching means stretching while moving. Usually the arm or leg swings several times through an arc of a range of motion. (See chapter 4 for examples of dynamic stretches.) Dynamic stretching stretches the muscle while the extremity is moving, so it is a more functional type of stretch with many variations. You can modify dynamic stretches in accordance with functional range of motion for the anticipated exercise program and in accordance with individual injury history and joint flexibility. Stretching should be done with warm muscles, so do a few minutes of gentle warm-up exercise (e.g., jogging for a runner) before stretching.

Measuring Your Fitness Level

Some people may wish to start an exercise program without first assessing their current fitness level. As noted, this approach is reasonable for most people, and just about everyone is better off exercising than not. However, assessing fitness at the outset of an exercise program can help to target activity to address fitness goals. Repeat assessments over the course of time may help to evaluate progress toward these goals and maintain exercise motivation. Ideally, an exercise program results in improvement in the parameters measured by these tests.

One important benefit of exercise is an increase in lean body mass. You can follow your progress by tracking your body mass index. Several changes occur in the body with an aerobic exercise program. The heart pumps blood and oxygen more effectively to the periphery, and the muscles become better able to extract oxygen and nutrients from the blood. You can measure the effect of these changes with an aerobic test. You can also follow strength and flexibility improvements as you continue an exercise program.

Body Mass Index

For most people starting an exercise program, body mass index (BMI) is a good indicator of how much fat, or adipose tissue, is present in the body. BMI is a number you can track to assess success in decreasing adipose tissue over time. It is calculated using the following equation:

BMI = [weight in pounds ÷ (height in inches × height in inches)] × 703

Weight may also be an acceptable parameter to follow, but BMI is easy to ascertain using the equation or from a BMI chart, and it is accepted as a more accurate marker for this important variable (see table 2.1). BMI

Table 2.1 Body Mass Index Values

To use this table, find your height in the left-hand column. Move across to your weight. The number at the top of the column is the BMI at that height and weight. Pounds have been rounded off.

BMI	19	20	21	22	23	24	25	26	27	28	29	30
Height (inches)	Body weight (pounds)											
58	91	96	100	105	110	115	119	124	129	134	138	143
59	94	99	104	109	114	119	124	128	133	138	143	148
60	97	102	107	112	118	123	128	133	138	143	148	153
61	100	106	111	116	122	127	132	137	143	148	153	158
62	104	109	115	120	126	131	136	142	147	153	158	164
63	107	113	118	124	130	135	141	146	152	158	163	169
64	110	116	122	128	134	140	145	151	157	163	169	174
65	114	120	126	132	138	144	150	156	162	168	174	180
66	118	124	130	136	142	148	155	161	167	173	179	186
67	121	127	134	140	146	153	159	166	172	178	185	191
68	125	131	138	144	151	158	164	171	177	184	190	197
69	128	135	142	149	155	162	169	176	182	189	196	203
70	132	139	146	153	160	167	174	181	188	195	202	209
71	136	143	150	157	165	172	179	186	193	200	208	215
72	140	147	154	162	169	177	184	191	199	206	213	221
73	144	151	159	166	174	182	189	197	204	212	219	227
74	148	155	163	171	179	186	194	202	210	218	225	233
75	152	160	168	176	184	192	200	208	216	224	232	240
76	156	164	172	180	189	197	205	213	221	230	238	246

BMI	31	32	33	34	35	36	37	38	39	40	41	42
58	148	153	158	162	167	172	177	181	186	191	196	201
59	153	158	163	168	173	178	183	188	193	198	203	208
60	158	163	168	174	179	184	189	194	199	204	209	215
61	164	169	174	180	185	190	195	201	206	211	217	222
62	169	175	180	186	191	196	202	207	213	218	224	229
63	175	180	186	191	197	203	208	214	220	225	231	237
64	180	186	192	197	204	209	215	221	227	232	238	244
65	186	192	198	204	210	216	222	228	234	240	246	252
66	192	198	204	210	216	223	229	235	241	247	253	260
67	198	204	211	217	223	230	236	242	249	255	261	268
68	203	210	216	223	230	236	243	249	256	262	269	276
69	209	216	223	230	236	243	250	257	263	270	277	284
70	216	222	229	236	243	250	257	264	271	278	285	292
71	222	229	236	243	250	257	265	272	279	286	293	301
72	228	235	242	250	258	265	272	279	287	294	302	309
73	235	242	250	257	265	272	280	288	295	302	310	318
74	241	249	256	264	272	280	287	295	303	311	319	326
75	248	256	264	272	279	287	295	303	311	319	327	335
76	254	263	271	279	287	295	304	312	320	328	336	344
BMI	43	44	45	46	47	48	49	50	51	52	53	54
58	205	210	215	220	224	229	234	239	244	248	253	258
59	212	217	222	227	232	237	242	247	252	257	262	267
60	220	225	230	235	240	245	250	255	261	266	271	276
61	227	232	238	243	248	254	259	264	269	275	280	285
62	235	240	246	251	256	262	267	273	278	284	289	295
63	242	248	254	259	265	270	278	282	287	293	299	304
64	250	256	262	267	273	279	285	291	296	302	308	314
65	258	264	270	276	282	288	294	300	306	312	318	324
66	266	272	278	284	291	297	303	309	315	322	328	334
67	274	280	287	293	299	306	312	319	325	331	338	344
68	282	289	295	302	308	315	322	328	335	341	348	354
69	291	297	304	311	318	324	331	338	345	351	358	365
70	299	306	313	320	327	334	341	348	355	362	369	376
71	308	315	322	329	338	343	351	358	365	372	379	386
72	316	324	331	338	346	353	361	368	375	383	390	397
73	325	333	340	348	355	363	371	378	386	393	401	408
74	334	342	350	358	365	373	381	389	396	404	412	420
75	343	351	359	367	375	383	391	399	407	415	423	431
76	353	361	369	377	385	394	402	410	418	426	435	443

Reprinted from the Centers for Disease Control and Prevention (CDC).

is a variable that changes slowly, even in a successful exercise program. It is probably reasonable to reevaluate BMI every 3 months or so. What matters is the long-term trend, not day-to-day fluctuations.

Aerobic Tests

You can measure aerobic capacity or aerobic fitness using one of several well-studied tests that will give you an accurate baseline for cardiovascular fitness. You can also repeat these tests after several months of an aerobic program to monitor changes in aerobic capacity. Your physician may recommend a maximal treadmill test to help make certain that no cardiovascular disease is present. All of these tests can estimate or measure $\dot{V}O_2max$, which is widely accepted as the truest measure of aerobic fitness. This value is "trainable"; that is, it increases as your fitness improves. Tables 2.2 and 2.3 list $\dot{V}O_2max$ values by age and sex. Many of these tests will also necessitate taking your pulse (see chapter 3).

Table 2.2   Percentile Values for $\dot{V}O_2max$ (ml/kg/min) in Men

	Age (years)				
Percentile	20-29 (N = 2,234)	30-39 (N = 11,158)	40-49 (N = 13,109)	50-59 (N = 5,641)	60+ (N = 1,244)
90	55.1	52.1	50.6	49.0	44.2
80	52.1	50.6	49.0	44.2	41.0
70	49.0	47.4	45.8	41.0	37.8
60	47.4	44.2	44.2	39.4	36.2
50	44.2	42.6	41.0	37.8	34.6
40	42.6	41.0	39.4	36.2	33.0
30	41.0	39.4	36.2	34.6	31.4
20	37.8	36.2	34.6	31.4	28.3
10	34.6	33.0	31.4	29.9	26.7

Data were obtained from the initial examination of apparently healthy men enrolled in the Aerobics Center Longitudinal Study (ACLS), 1970 to 2002. The study population for the data set was predominantly Caucasian and college educated. Maximal treadmill exercise tests were administered using a modified Balke protocol. Maximal oxygen uptake was estimated from the final treadmill speed and grade using the current ACSM equations found in the seventh edition of the *Guidelines.* The data are provided courtesy of the ACLS investigators, The Cooper Institute, Dallas, TX. The ACLS is supported in part by a grant from the National Institute on Aging (AG06945), SN Blair, Principal Investigator. The following may be used as descriptors for the percentile rankings: well above average (90), above average (70), average (50), below average (30), and well below average (10).

Adapted, by permission, from ACSM, 2006, *ACSM's guidelines for exercise testing and prescription,* 7th ed. (Philadelphia, PA: Lippincott, Williams & Wilkins), 79.

Table 2.3   Percentile Values for $\dot{V}O_2$max (ml/kg/min) in Women

Percentile	Age (years)				
	20-29 (N = 1,223)	30-39 (N = 3,895)	40-49 (N = 4,001)	50-59 (N = 2,032)	60+ (N = 465)
90	49.0	45.8	42.6	37.8	34.6
80	44.2	41.0	39.4	34.6	33.0
70	41.0	39.4	36.2	33.0	31.4
60	39.4	36.2	34.6	31.4	28.3
50	37.8	34.6	33.0	29.9	26.7
40	36.2	33.0	31.4	28.3	25.1
30	33.0	31.4	29.9	26.7	23.5
20	31.4	29.9	28.3	25.1	21.9
10	28.3	26.7	25.1	21.9	20.3

Data were obtained from the initial examination of apparently healthy women enrolled in the Aerobics Center Longitudinal Study (ACLS), 1970 to 2002. The study population for the data set was predominantly Caucasian and college educated. Maximal treadmill exercise tests were administered using a modified Balke protocol. Maximal oxygen uptake was estimated from the final treadmill speed and grade using the current ACSM equations found in the seventh edition of the *Guidelines*. The data are provided courtesy of the ACLS investigators, The Cooper Institute, Dallas, TX. The ACLS is supported in part by a grant from the National Institute on Aging (AG06945), SN Blair, Principal Investigator. The following may be used as descriptors for the percentile rankings: well above average (90), above average (70), average (50), below average (30), and well below average (10).

Adapted, by permission, from ACSM, 2006, *ACSM's guidelines for exercise testing and prescription*, 7th ed. (Philadelphia, PA: Lippincott, Williams & Wilkins), 79.

Rockport Walking Test

This test has been evaluated and validated on healthy adults. It is easy to perform and replicate. It involves timing yourself while walking 1 mile and taking your pulse afterward. You can repeat the test to monitor fitness progress.

To perform the test, you will need a 400-meter track or any other measured course, a stopwatch, and a weight scale. Follow these steps:

1. Measure body weight to the nearest pound.
2. Walk 1 mile as quickly as possible, noting your total time to complete the mile.
3. At the end of the mile, immediately take your pulse for 10 seconds. Multiply this number by 6 to obtain your heart rate in beats per minute (bpm).
4. Convert your walking time from minutes and seconds to minute units. To calculate minute units, divide the number of seconds by

60 to get a fraction (round up to the nearest hundredth). Thus, a walking time of 15 minutes and 37 seconds would become 15 + (37/60) = 15.62.

5. Calculate your estimated maximal oxygen consumption ($\dot{V}O_2$max) using the following formula. Then use table 2.2 or 2.3 on page 26 or 27 to determine your fitness classification.

$$\dot{V}O_2\text{max in ml/kg/min} = 132.853 - (.0769 \times W) - (.3877 \times A) + (6.315 \times S) - (3.2649 \times T) - (.1565 \times HR)$$

W = weight in pounds

A = age in years

S = sex (0 = female; 1 = male)

T = total converted time in minutes

HR = heart rate in bpm for 1-mile walk

For example, a 49-year-old female who weighs 145 pounds has a walk time of 16 minutes and 42 seconds, and her 10-second pulse is 23. The calculation would look like this:

$$T = 16 + 42/60 = 16.7$$
$$HR = 23 \times 6 = 138 \text{ bpm}$$
$$\dot{V}O_2\text{max} = 132.853 - (0.0769 \times 145) - (0.3877 \times 49) + (6.315 \times 0) - (3.2649 \times 16.7) - (0.1565 \times 138)$$
$$= 132.853 - 11.1505 - 18.9973 + 0 - 54.52383 - 21.597$$
$$\dot{V}O_2\text{max} = 26.6 \text{ ml/kg/min}$$

Adapted, by permission, from G.M. Kline, J.P. Porcari, R. Hintermeister, P.S. Freedson, A. Ward, R.F. McCarron, J. Ross, and J.M. Rippe, 1987, "Estimation of $\dot{V}O_2$max from a one mile track walk, gender, age, and body weight," *Medicine and Science in Sports and Exercise* 19: 253-59.

Submaximal Bicycle Test

The Åstrand-Rhyming cycling test has been well validated on healthy subjects. It is also fairly easy to perform. You need a stationary bicycle with resistance levels that can be set between 300 and 900 kilogram-meters per minute (kpm), a stopwatch, and a weight scale. The test involves cycling at a given resistance at 50 revolutions per minute (rpm). Then the pulse is taken at 1-minute intervals over 6 minutes. It may be helpful to do this test with a partner who can monitor your pulse rate, because it involves taking your pulse during exercise. Your oxygen consumption is then calculated using a nomogram chart that is adjusted for age. Here are the steps to take for this assessment:

1. Measure your body weight to the nearest pound and convert to kilograms (weight in pounds divided by 2.2046).

2. Adjust the bicycle seat; at the bottom of the pedal revolution, your knee should be almost completely straight.

3. Start pedaling, increasing speed to 50 rpm. Maintaining this speed throughout the test, increase the resistance to the recommended level (consider your age and health; if you are older or in poorer health, select the lower of the two levels):

	Females	Males
Unconditioned	300 or 450 kpm	300 or 600 kpm
Conditioned	450 or 600 kpm	600 or 900 kpm

4. Start the stopwatch, continuing pedal cadence for 6 minutes. Check your heart rate for the last 10 seconds of each minute. Convert each 10-second count to heart rate in bpm by multiplying each count by 6.

5. If minutes 5 and 6 are within 5 beats of each other, average them to get your test heart rate. Otherwise, continue for a few minutes until they are within 5 beats of each other. If your heart rate continues to increase greatly after minute 6, stop the test and rest for approximately 15 minutes. You may then perform the test again at the next lower workload. Your final average heart rate should be from 120 to 140 bpm for the lower workloads and from 120 to 170 for the higher workloads.

6. Using the final averaged heart rate, find your $\dot{V}O_2$max (l/min) in table 2.4. Then correct for age by multiplying this value by your age correction factor from table 2.5.

7. To find $\dot{V}O_2$max in ml/kg/min, complete the following calculations:

$$\dot{V}O_2\text{max in ml/kg/min} = (l/min \times 1{,}000) \div \text{Weight (kg)}$$

8. Using the oxygen consumption value, find your fitness classification in table 2.2 or 2.3.

For example, a 67-year-old male, unconditioned and with a weight of 195 pounds, completes the test at 300 kpm, with an average heart rate of 132 bpm. The calculation would look like this:

$$\dot{V}O_2\text{max (l/min)} = 1.8$$

$$\dot{V}O_2\text{max (l/min) age corrected} = .65 \times 1.8 = 1.17$$

$$\text{Weight} = 88.5 \text{ kg}$$

$$\dot{V}O_2\text{max in ml/kg/min} = (1.17 \times 1{,}000) \div 88.5 = 13.2 \text{ ml/kg/min}$$

Adapted, by permission, from I. Astrand, 1960, "Aerobic work capacity in men and women with special reference to age," *Acta Physiologica Scandinavica* 49(Suppl 169): 1-92.

Table 2.4 Åstrand-Rhyming Bicycle Test—Oxygen Consumption Rates Based on Workload and Heart Rate

Heart rate	Workload for men					Workload for women				
	300	600	900	1200	1500	300	450	600	750	900
120	2.2	3.4	4.8			2.6	3.4	4.1	4.8	
121	2.2	3.4	4.7			2.5	3.3	4.0	4.8	
122	2.2	3.4	4.6			2.5	3.2	3.9	4.7	
123	2.1	3.4	4.6			2.4	3.1	3.9	4.6	
124	2.1	3.3	4.5	6.0		2.4	3.1	3.8	4.5	
125	2.0	3.2	4.4	5.9		2.3	3.0	3.7	4.4	
126	2.0	3.2	4.4	5.8		2.3	3.0	3.6	4.3	
127	2.0	3.1	4.3	5.7		2.2	2.9	3.5	4.2	
128	2.0	3.1	4.2	5.6		2.2	2.8	3.5	4.2	4.8
129	1.9	3.0	4.2	5.6		2.2	2.8	3.4	4.1	4.8
130	1.9	3.0	4.1	5.5		2.1	2.7	3.4	4.0	4.7
131	1.9	2.9	4.0	5.4		2.1	2.7	3.4	4.0	4.6
132	1.8	2.9	4.0	5.3		2.0	2.7	3.3	3.9	4.5
133	1.8	2.8	3.9	5.3		2.0	2.6	3.2	3.8	4.4
134	1.8	2.8	3.9	5.2		2.0	2.6	3.2	3.8	4.4
135	1.7	2.8	3.8	5.1		2.0	2.6	3.1	3.7	4.3
136	1.7	2.7	3.8	5.0		1.9	2.5	3.1	3.6	4.2
137	1.7	2.7	3.7	5.0		1.9	2.5	3.0	3.6	4.2
138	1.6	2.7	3.7	4.9		1.8	2.4	3.0	3.5	4.1
139	1.6	2.6	3.6	4.8		1.8	2.4	2.9	3.5	4.0
140	1.6	2.6	3.6	4.8	6.0	1.8	2.4	2.8	3.4	4.0
141		2.6	3.5	4.7	5.9	1.8	2.3	2.8	3.4	3.9
142		2.5	3.5	4.6	5.8	1.7	2.3	2.8	3.3	3.9
143		2.5	3.4	4.6	5.7	1.7	2.2	2.7	3.3	3.8
144		2.5	3.4	4.5	5.7	1.7	2.2	2.7	3.2	3.8
145		2.4	3.4	4.5	5.6	1.6	2.2	2.7	3.2	3.7
146		2.4	3.3	4.4	5.6	1.6	2.2	2.6	3.2	3.7
147		2.4	3.3	4.4	5.5	1.6	2.1	2.6	3.1	3.6
148		2.4	3.2	4.3	5.4	1.6	2.1	2.6	3.1	3.6
149		2.3	3.2	4.3	5.4		2.1	2.6	3.0	3.5
150		2.3	3.2	4.2	5.3		2.0	2.5	3.0	3.5
151		2.3	3.1	4.2	5.2		2.0	2.5	3.0	3.4
152		2.3	3.1	4.1	5.2		2.0	2.5	2.9	3.4
153		2.2	3.0	4.1	5.1		2.0	2.4	2.9	3.3
154		2.2	3.0	4.0	5.1		2.0	2.4	2.8	3.3
155		2.2	3.0	4.0	5.0		1.9	2.4	2.8	3.2
156		2.2	2.9	4.0	5.0		1.9	2.3	2.8	3.2
157		2.1	2.9	3.9	4.9		1.9	2.3	2.7	3.2
158		2.1	2.9	3.9	4.9		1.8	2.3	2.7	3.1

Heart rate	Workload for men					Workload for women				
	300	600	900	1200	1500	300	450	600	750	900
159		2.1	2.8	3.8	4.8		1.8	2.2	2.7	3.1
160		2.1	2.8	3.8	4.8		1.8	2.2	2.6	3.0
161		2.0	2.8	3.7	4.7		1.8	2.2	2.6	3.0
162		2.0	2.8	3.7	4.6		1.8	2.2	2.6	3.0
163		2.0	2.8	3.7	4.6		1.7	2.2	2.6	2.9
164		2.0	2.7	3.6	4.5		1.7	2.1	2.5	2.9
165		2.0	2.7	3.6	4.5		1.7	2.1	2.5	2.9
166		1.9	2.7	3.6	4.5		1.7	2.1	2.5	2.8
167		1.9	2.6	3.5	4.4		1.6	2.1	2.4	2.8
168		1.9	2.6	3.5	4.4		1.6	2.0	2.4	2.8
169		1.9	2.6	3.5	4.3		1.6	2.0	2.4	2.8
170		1.8	2.6	3.4	4.3		1.6	2.0	2.4	2.7

Reprinted, by permission, from I. Astrand, 1960, "Aerobic work capacity in men and women with special reference to age," *Acta Physiologica Scandinavica* 49(Suppl 169): 1-92.

Table 2.5 Age Correction Factors

Age	Correction factor	Age	Correction factor
20	1.05	43	.800
21	1.04	44	.790
22	1.03	45	.780
23	1.02	46	.774
24	1.01	47	.768
25	1.00	48	.762
26	.987	49	.756
27	.974	50	.750
28	.961	51	.742
29	.948	52	.734
30	.935	53	.726
31	.922	54	.718
32	.909	55	.710
33	.896	56	.704
34	.883	57	.698
35	.870	58	.692
36	.862	59	.686
37	.854	60	.680
38	.846	61	.674
39	.838	62	.668
40	.830	63	.662
41	.820	64	.656
42	.810	65	.650

Reprinted, by permission, from I. Astrand, 1960, "Aerobic work capacity in men and women with special reference to age," *Acta Physiologica Scandinavica* 49(Suppl 169): 1-92.

Time Trials

If you run, cycle, or swim regularly, a good measure of sport-specific aerobic fitness may be a time trial. Every so often, time yourself over the same distance (e.g., a 1-mile run) to assess your improvement. People who view their training as a means to an end in the form of endurance competition can use their time in their chosen event as an indicator of the effectiveness of their training program. For instance, an Olympic-distance triathlon time that drops from 2 hours, 25 minutes to 2 hours, 15 minutes would demonstrate an improvement in aerobic fitness as well as validate the success of that competitor's training program.

Strength Testing

The traditional measure of strength is the maximal amount of weight that can be lifted one time. This 1-repetition maximal lift (1RM) is the test of strength in Olympic weightlifting. It is a reasonable standard for adult competitive weightlifters who have been in training for some time. However, the 1RM may have an unnecessarily high risk of injury in individuals who are starting a strength program for fitness. A good functional test for most exercisers is to monitor the amount of weight that they can lift in a given exercise for 8 repetitions with correct technique. For instance, assume that a person may be able to do 8 triceps curls with 6 plates of weighted resistance upon starting a training program. Then that person does a resistance program twice a week over 6 months. If at that time the individual can do 8 triceps curls with 10 plates, elbow extension strength has improved. More functional tests are available for individuals as they begin a resistance program. Following are two tests to measure strength in the arm, trunk, and abdominal muscles.

Push-Up Test

The push-up test is a good measure of arm and trunk strength. To perform this test, follow this procedure:

1. Lie facedown on the ground and position your hands by your shoulders (palms down). Men will keep legs straight, with their feet as the lower contact point, while women will bend their knees to 90 degrees, using the knees as the lower contact point.
2. Push up until arms are fully extended, then lower the body toward the floor. When lowered, the chest should be no higher than 4 inches (a fist width) from the floor, but it should not touch the floor between push-ups.
3. Your back must remain straight throughout the push-up.
4. Count the number of push-ups you complete without stopping (you have no time limit).
5. Calculate your fitness level using table 2.6.

Table 2.6 Fitness Classifications for Push-Up Test Scores

	Age									
Category	**20-29**		**30-39**		**40-49**		**50-59**		**60-69**	
Gender	**M**	**F**	**M**	**F**	**M**	**F**	**M**	**F**	**M**	**F**
Excellent	36	30	30	27	25	24	21	21	18	17
Very good	35	29	29	26	24	23	20	20	17	16
	29	21	22	20	17	15	13	11	11	12
Good	28	20	21	19	16	14	12	10	10	11
	22	15	17	13	13	11	10	7	8	5
Fair	21	14	16	12	12	10	9	6	7	4
	17	10	12	8	10	5	7	2	5	2
Needs improvement	16	9	11	7	9	4	6	1	4	1

Source: The Canadian Physical Activity, Fitness & Lifestyle Approach: CSEP-Health & Fitness Program's Health-Related Appraisal and Counseling Strategy. 3rd Edition © 2003. Reprinted with permission of the Canadian Society for Exercise Physiology.

Curl-Up Test

Abdominal muscle strength is usually addressed in a resistance program. Physical therapists refer to the trunk muscles as "the core." They have realized in recent years that core strength and stability are essential to minimize the risk of injury in many types of athletic activity. Abdominal muscles are important contributors to core stability. A good test of abdominal strength is the timed curl-up test. To perform this test, follow these steps:

1. Lie on your back with your knees bent to approximately 100 degrees (feet flat on the floor). Cross your arms over your chest, putting each hand on the opposite shoulder.
2. Raise your head off the floor, with chin on chest, and bring your body to an upright position, then lower yourself back to the floor.
3. Complete as many repetitions as possible in a 1-minute period, and count the number of complete curl-ups.
4. Figure your fitness rating from table 2.7.

Table 2.7   Fitness Classifications for Curl-Up Test Scores

Category	Age									
	20-29		30-39		40-49		50-59		60-69	
Gender	M	F	M	F	M	F	M	F	M	F
Excellent	25	25	25	25	25	25	25	25	25	25
Very good	24	24	24	24	24	24	24	24	24	24
	21	18	18	19	18	19	17	19	16	17
Good	20	17	17	18	17	18	16	18	15	16
	16	14	15	10	13	11	11	10	11	8
Fair	15	13	14	9	12	10	10	9	10	7
	11	5	11	6	6	4	8	6	6	3
Needs improvement	10	4	10	5	5	3	7	5	5	2

Source: The Canadian Physical Activity, Fitness & Lifestyle Approach: CSEP-Health & Fitness Program's Health-Related Appraisal and Counseling Strategy. 3rd Edition © 2003. Reprinted with permission of the Canadian Society for Exercise Physiology.

Flexibility Tests

A good measure of flexibility is the sit-and-reach test. To perform this test, you will need a yardstick and a piece of tape. Mark the yardstick at 15 inches with the tape. Sit on the floor with your legs in front of you, feet a little less than shoulder-width apart. Place the yardstick between your legs, with the 15-inch mark at your heels and the zero end toward your body. Placing one hand on top of the other and keeping your back straight, lean forward as far as possible. Try to keep your knees as straight as possible and your hands together (don't reach farther forward with one or the other). Don't hold your breath while stretching. Have a partner mark how far down the yardstick you reached, and find your score in table 2.8.

If you are in the poor category or below, you should incorporate dynamic stretches into your program. Dynamic or functional stretches are discussed in more detail in chapter 4. These stretches involve elongating a muscle as far as it will go, then rotating the body part served by that muscle and moving it from side to side. This sort of flexibility activity more closely approximates the stresses placed on muscles during activity. The core muscles support the pelvis from above and below. They include the low back, abdominal, and hip muscles. Maintaining strength and flexibility in these muscles allows the exerciser to maintain a stable core, which can help to prevent injury.

Table 2.8 **Percentiles for Sit-and-Reach Test Scores**

	Age											
Percentile	**18-25**		**26-35**		**36-45**		**46-55**		**56-65**		**Over 65**	
Gender	**M**	**F**	**M**	**F**	**M**	**F**	**M**	**F**	**M**	**F**	**M**	**F**
90	22	24	21	23	21	22	19	21	17	20	17	20
80	20	22	19	21	19	21	17	20	15	19	15	18
70	19	21	17	20	17	19	15	18	13	17	13	17
60	18	20	17	20	16	18	14	17	13	16	12	17
50	17	19	15	19	15	17	13	16	11	15	10	15
40	15	18	14	17	13	16	11	14	9	14	9	14
30	14	17	13	16	13	15	10	14	9	13	8	13
20	13	16	11	15	11	14	9	12	7	11	7	11
10	11	14	9	13	7	12	6	10	5	9	4	9

Adapted from *YMCA Fitness Testing and Assessment Manual*, 4th edition, 2000, with permission of YMCA of the USA, 101 N. Wacker Drive, Chicago, IL 60606.

Warm-Up and Cool-Down

As muscles are used their blood flow increases and they become warmer. In animal studies, warm muscle has greater elasticity and stretches farther before it ruptures. So, gently work the same muscles that will be used in a training session over 5 to 10 minutes at the beginning of that session. Doing so may decrease the chance of muscle pain or injury. Often people stretch just after their initial warm-up. Again, dynamic stretching is the most beneficial type of stretching.

You can also use warm-up to enhance tolerance of exercise activity and decrease the likelihood of allergic symptoms. For example, a track and field athlete in the mile run has exercise-induced asthma (EIA). If she warms up 30 minutes before her event by running for 15 minutes at a pace of 8 minutes per mile, she will be much more likely to complete her mile in 4 minutes, 45 seconds without symptoms. Most athletes with EIA will perform best if they use their warm-up to enhance tolerance *and* take their inhaler. Two puffs on the albuterol inhaler should be taken 15 minutes before the start of the warm-up.

For 5 to 15 minutes at the end of a workout, it is a good idea to use the muscles that were exercised in a less strenuous fashion as a cool-down to conclude the exercise session. It might be useful to lightly stretch these muscles because muscles may functionally contract as they adapt to the range of motion needed for a given activity.

Allergic symptoms, especially wheezing and coughing of asthma, may be more likely to occur during cool-down than during exercise itself. An albuterol inhaler must be readily available before, during, and after a workout. If asthmatic symptoms occur, two puffs of albuterol should be taken as a "rescue" medication, repeating this dose in 20 minutes if needed. Having to use an inhaler in this fashion more than twice a week usually means you need better prophylaxis. It may indicate a need for either another medication for EIA before exercise, or better control of the inflammatory component of the baseline asthma.

Monitoring Your Exercise Progress

Just as it is important to write down goals at the outset, it is helpful to monitor progress toward those goals as a result of exercise. A good measure of cardiovascular fitness for most people is their resting pulse. In patients who are not taking medications that affect heart rate, a good pulse is 72, parameters to follow. In general, an average resting pulse over 85 indicates poor fitness. Marathon runners may have a resting pulse rate of 40 or even less. (See Establishing Individual Exercise Intensity in chapter 3.)

If weight loss is an exercise goal, the only way to monitor it is to step on the scale and check your weight. It is probably not necessary to do this any more frequently than every 2 weeks. Remember that the weight trend is what is important. Everyone who has successfully completed and maintained a weight loss program has had episodes where they gained weight *during the program*. If weight gain occurs, it does not mean that you have no willpower or that exercise is pointless and that you should quit your program. It's an expected part of the process. Indeed, it is true that muscle weighs more than fat. As an individual becomes more fit, lean body mass increases. With strength training, muscle hypertrophies result in a net increase in weight even as the amount of fat in the body decreases.

One option to accurately monitor this process is to follow lean body weight or percent body fat over time. An accurate method for this measurement is underwater weighing. Unfortunately, it is not a convenient method for most people to access. Some exercise physiologists can give an accurate assessment of percent body fat using skinfold caliper measurements.

As noted, strength can be monitored by carefully cataloguing repetitions, sets, and weight lifted over time. As greater amounts of weight can be lifted for more repetitions, strength gains are occurring.

Hydration

Individuals who have an allergic response during exercise are generally more likely to lose more body water during exercise. This is particularly true for respiratory allergies. Inflammation of the mucous membranes of the mouth and airways results in increased fluid loss through these surfaces during an allergic response. Water is the most important nutrient for all exercisers. Make sure that you do not start off an exercise session feeling thirsty or with a dry mouth. In fact, if you feel thirsty you may already be dehydrated. Most individuals lose 5 percent of their body water before they sense a feeling of thirst. Strenuous exercise can have serious medical consequences in the setting of dehydration. Problems may include kidney failure and even death.

People may sweat more than a liter of fluid during strenuous exercise in conditions of high heat and humidity. Drinking a liter of fluid for each hour of exercise in these conditions is probably a good idea. For exercise duration of an hour or less, water is the optimum fluid replacement drink. For longer durations, a sports drink that replaces electrolytes (especially sodium) and carbohydrates may be a good choice. One approximate measure of hydration status is color of one's urine. Brownish-yellow indicates concentrated urine consistent with dehydration. Clear white urine may indicate overhydration, which may put a person at risk for severe medical problems such as hyponatremia (low sodium in the bloodstream) during exercise. Light yellow, the color of lemonade, indicates appropriate hydration for exercise.

Sample Program

So what would a new exercise program for an overweight person with asthma look like? A full set of sample programs to address fitness goals appears in later chapters, but here is a quick example of what a program, including progress assessments and adjustments, might look like:

Our sample patient is Joe, a 47-year-old man who was diagnosed with asthma as a child. Currently he is in the Green zone of his asthma action plan for his peak flow on Advair Diskus 250/50 (one inhalation, twice daily). He has an albuterol rescue inhaler that he has not needed for 4 months. He is 5 feet, 8 inches tall and weighs 198 pounds. So his BMI is 30, which puts him in the obese range. His 1-mile walk test estimated his $\dot{V}O_2$max at 33, which puts him in the fair range. He can do 24 push-ups, so he has good upper body strength. His sit-and-reach flexibility is poor.

Joe wants to initiate a walking program with a primary goal of eventually losing 40 pounds. This weight loss would improve his BMI to 24, the upper end of the normal range. His secondary goal is to improve his aerobic fitness. He has no history of arthritis or previous surgery in his knees, ankles, or hips, so walking is a reasonable exercise choice for him. Eventually, running may become a viable option. He feels that his busy work schedule as an accountant allows him 1 hour for exercise on 3 days a week and half an hour for exercise on 3 other days a week.

Here is his exercise prescription:

First 3 Months: Starting a Program

For all sessions: 15 minutes before each session, 2 puffs albuterol to prevent exercise-induced asthma symptoms	
Warm-up	Slow walk for 4 minutes.
	1 minute of dynamic quadriceps, hamstring, and gastrocnemius stretches.
60-minute sessions	Walk at a pace where sweating occurs after 10 minutes.
	Maintain this pace for 50 minutes.
	Cool down with 5 minutes of walking at a slower pace combined with the same dynamic stretches as noted.
30-minute sessions	Walk at a pace where sweating occurs after 6 to 8 minutes.
	Maintain this pace for 20 minutes.
	Cool down with 5 minutes of walking at a slower pace combined with the same dynamic stretches as noted.

He has elected to focus on his goals and has not addressed strength training at the outset. His strength assessment was in the good range, so this initial program was a reasonable one. To get the greatest possible benefit from his 30-minute exercise sessions, he has chosen to exercise at a greater estimated intensity on these days.

After 3 months he weighs 186 (BMI 28), and his resting pulse has dropped from 85 to 75. He has become interested in following his fitness progress more closely and adding in some strength training. He has made his fitness a high priority and come to the realization that he can free up an hour for exercise on 6 days each week. He has decided to join a gym with cardiovascular and resistance equipment to help him attain his goals. He thinks that a circuit program may be the easiest type of exercise for him to stick with over time.

After 3 Months: Maintenance Program

For all sessions: 15 minutes before each session, 2 puffs albuterol to prevent exercise-induced asthma symptoms	
First 15 minutes	Warm-up: 3 minutes on a stationary bicycle at an easy level followed by 2 minutes of dynamic stretching of the trunk, legs, and arms
	Cardiovascular: 10 minutes on a stepper at a pulse rate of 144 (70 percent of maximal heart rate)
Last 15 minutes	Cardiovascular: 10 minutes on a treadmill at a pulse of 144
	Cool-down: 5 minutes, same as warm-up

This leaves 30 minutes in the middle of each workout session for resistance training. For circuit training to be successful, Joe should move rapidly from one exercise to the next. He should try to wait no longer than 30 seconds between sets. He will try to keep his pulse between 100 and 140 beats per minute.

Days 1, 3, 5: Trunk and legs	50 crunches for upper abdomen
	20 lumbar (low back) extensions
	15 left and 15 right side bends with 10-pound weight for abdominal obliques
	2 sets of 12 hip adduction
	2 sets of 12 hip abduction
	2 sets of 12 leg presses
	2 sets of 12 quadriceps extensions
	2 sets of 12 toe raises
	30 leg lifts for lower abdomen
Days 2, 4, 6: Arms	2 sets of 12 seated rows for rhomboids—upper back
	2 sets of 12 bench presses—pectoralis muscles
	2 sets of 12 latissimus pull-downs
	2 sets of 12 overhead presses
	2 sets of 12 shoulder shrugs
	2 sets of 12 deltoid raises
	2 sets of 12 biceps curls
	2 sets of 12 triceps extensions

If his resistance exercises do not fill the entire 30 minutes, he can do an extra set of each. Another option would be adding a few minutes on to one or both cardiovascular exercise sessions.

Sticking With It

Certain aspects of any behavior make that behavior more likely to occur. Humans are social animals, and exercise that is done with a group is more likely to be maintained over time. At our hospital's fitness center, a group of men started exercising together weekday mornings several years ago. Then they began getting together for lunch afterward and called themselves "The Lunch Bunch." For them, exercising with the group has become a social outlet, and the gentle ribbing they get from other members of the Bunch if they don't show up has become a powerful motivator for consistent exercise behavior. Even exercise with a single partner increases the likelihood that the behavior will persist.

Some people get personal satisfaction from the exact same exercise regimen 6 days a week for many years; others find that their exercise routine becomes stale with repetition. Changing things up may be the key to maintaining motivation. Any cardiovascular activity that can be done at the desired intensity for the desired amount of time may be substituted without a decrease in the effectiveness of the program. A 1-hour bike ride with friends may give you the same cardiovascular overload as a half-hour run.

A program to maximize muscle endurance with resistance exercise (e.g., 15 repetitions of each exercise) may be motivating for an exerciser over several weeks. Over the next few weeks, it can be alternated with a program to maximize strength and muscle hypertrophy (e.g., 8 repetitions).

Some people elect to combine strength and cardiovascular exercise to obtain the benefits of both in a shorter time. This is the concept of circuit training. A few minutes of aerobic exercise usually start and end a circuit. The individual goes quickly from one set of resistance exercises to another, maintaining an elevated heart rate throughout the circuit. Typically arm and leg resistance exercises are alternated over a period of 30 to 60 minutes. Several national chains of exercise centers offer circuit exercise programs.

For many exercisers, increasing the variety in their program helps to keep them interested and motivated, so cross-training is an attractive option. Cross-training may also decrease the likelihood of overuse injury. Cycling or swimming, for instance, lessens the impact forces of exercise and decreases the risk of stress fracture relative to running.

Some people need a goal to justify their ongoing exercise behavior. For me the activity that keeps me going is playing volleyball in the summer on the beach at Lake Michigan. I know the level of fitness necessary to cover half the court playing beach doubles. This reinforces my regular cardiovascular and resistance exercise circuit program during the rest of the year.

A final consideration in the maintenance of exercise behavior is reevaluating and resetting goals over time. Injuries, illnesses or home or work responsibilities may necessitate scaling back goals for the short term. As fitness improves, previously unattainable goals may become attainable.

Summary

The benefits of exercise are the same for people with allergies as they are for anyone else. There really is no reason why people with allergies should not be able to attain all of these benefits by pursuing whatever fitness goals they desire. It is essential that the appropriate medication be taken in a timely fashion to avoid allergy symptoms during exercise. Allergy patients need to be aware of triggers for their symptoms and either avoid them or take steps to minimize their impact on exercise activity. Similarly, the important components of an exercise program are no different for people with allergies than they are for all exercisers. For a program to be effective, you must first ascertain your fitness goals. Then you can build an exercise program around these goals.

See your physician first if you are starting a new program and you have two or more cardiac risk factors. Assess your fitness level before starting and periodically as you pursue your fitness goals. To achieve a training effect, you should exercise between 3 and 6 times a week for between 30 and 60 minutes. Aerobic activity should be done at an intensity level where sweating occurs. Strength training and dynamic flexibility activity should be incorporated into your program. Remember, a training effect can be lost in a matter of weeks, so it is essential to keep your program going once you have started. The following chapters will provide specific guidelines for tailoring your cardiovascular, strength, and flexibility programs to your needs and fitness levels so that you can overcome the obstacle your allergies present to exercising.

ACTION PLAN:
DESIGNING AN EXERCISE PROGRAM

☐ Set realistic, attainable goals. Identify short-term and long-term goals.

☐ Remember exercise guidelines:

- aerobic activity 3 to 6 times weekly for 20 to 60 minutes
- strength training 3 times weekly
- dynamic stretching before and after each exercise session.

☐ Follow your body mass index every 3 months to evaluate fat loss (or gain).

☐ Consider conducting a fitness evaluation when you start your exercise program, using the tests given in this chapter. Repeat this evaluation every 6 to 12 months to follow your fitness level.

☐ Have fun!

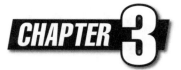

TARGETING ASTHMA THROUGH AEROBIC EXERCISE

Matthew J. Brandon

Whether augmenting or fine-tuning your exercise routine, adding aerobic exercise can improve your asthma symptoms, and you can take steps to ensure your allergies will not interfere with your new or modified exercise program. Numerous studies confirm the benefits of aerobic exercise in common medical conditions such as diabetes mellitus, heart disease, and arthritis. More than 40 years ago exercise was believed to increase risk of asthma severity. Today ample evidence shows that adding an aerobic exercise program can help people who have asthma. In fact, lack of physical activity in our society may correlate with an increased prevalence of asthma and allergy. Rasmussen et al. (2000) followed 750 children over 10 to 11 years and found a higher incidence of adolescent asthma in those children engaging in less physical activity. A study of twins by Huovinen et al. (2001) demonstrated less risk of developing asthma in the more physically active twin. Except in a few rare conditions, which will be discussed later, exercise does not cause allergies. However, someone with known allergies starting an aerobic exercise program requires special attention.

This chapter should serve as a guide for starting an aerobic exercise program but in no way is intended to replace the expert opinion of your personal physician. Always consider consulting your physician before starting a new exercise program.

Benefits of Aerobic Exercise

Several types of aerobic exercise exist, including but not limited to running or jogging, walking, cycling, and swimming. The benefits of aerobic exercise are multiple and include improved cardiovascular health, decreased blood pressure, weight reduction, improved respiratory performance, improved psychiatric health, less arthritic joint pain, favorable blood sugar and lipids, better sleep, and better cognitive function. Aerobic exercises include activities that require oxygen to produce energy in working muscles. These rhythmic, repetitive activities must be performed with adequate intensity, frequency, and duration in order to improve fitness. To meet the body's demand for energy, the heart, lungs, and circulatory system must work together to deliver the oxygen the body needs. These systems adapt to the increased demand by becoming more efficient at supplying energy and removing metabolic waste products.

It is well documented that aerobic exercise can improve and prevent problems such as cardiovascular disease, osteoarthritis, diabetes, hypertension, and hypercholesterolemia (U.S. Dept. of Health and Human Services 1996, Minor et al. 1989, Wei et al. 1999, Knowler et al. 2002, Krause et al. 2002). The adaptive physiologic changes in your cardiovascular system to aerobic exercise tend to be greater than adaptations to nonaerobic exercise. Benefits such as flexibility and muscle strength are to be gained from nonaerobic exercise, but cardiovascular and respiratory benefits are less pronounced. The rhythmic, repetitive movements of aerobic exercise are ideally suited to improving cardiovascular and respiratory function. Several physiologic changes occur in the body with aerobic exercise. To detail every advantageous physiologic change associated with aerobic exercise is beyond the scope of this chapter. However, the chapter details the positive effects aerobic exercise creates with respect to asthma (pulmonary function) and allergy (immunologic function).

You should not fear exercise if you currently have asthma, exercise-induced asthma (EIA), allergic rhinitis, or other physical allergies. In fact, the American Thoracic Society (ATS) and the American College of Sports Medicine (ACSM) have endorsed a prescription for aerobic exercise for all asthma patients (ACSM 2005). Further, it is becoming more apparent that a sedentary lifestyle has played a large role in the ever-increasing prevalence of asthma. Obesity has also been implicated in the rising prevalence of asthma. Logic would state that an exercise program may prevent the vicious cycle of inactivity and obesity to improve asthma symptoms. Medical literature for the past two decades has endorsed aerobic exercise conditioning as an adjunct to medical treatment. The message is overwhelming: It is safe for you, and it is recommended that you incorporate aerobic exercise into your routine.

By now you know it is safe for you to add jogging or running, walking, swimming, or cycling to your current exercise regimen. You're probably curious why aerobic exercise is so beneficial for asthma and EIA. Regardless of the aerobic exercise you choose, you should notice fewer wheezing episodes, diminished wheezing intensity, improved quality of life, reduction in medication use, fewer emergency visits, improved exercise or sport performance, and increased participation in physical activity. These findings have been confirmed in the following literature reviews: Orenstein (2002), Satta (2000), and Clark (1993). It should be noted that the majority of published studies relating to pulmonary performance and exercise prescription are related to chronic obstructive pulmonary disease (COPD) and emphysema. However, there is ample evidence published regarding asthma and EIA. You may have encountered many people with asthma who have avoided exercise because of difficulty with performance. This difficulty is generally a result of inactivity and not necessarily related to the severity of asthma. To that end, a survey of the 1984 Olympic athletes revealed that a large percentage of athletes with asthma not only participated but often won medals as well. Exercise will not cure you of asthma, but an aerobic exercise prescription under the guidance of a physician will improve your ability to be physically active.

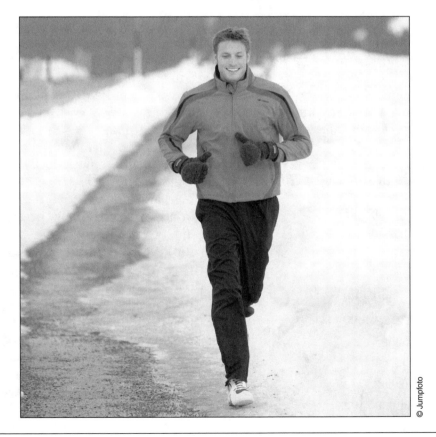

Physical activity and exercise are important parts of a strategy to combat obesity, thus helping to improve asthma symptoms.

Although aerobic exercise has proven beneficial for asthma and EIA, no one has proven clear benefit with regard to seasonal or physical allergies. Although evidence suggests that modest exercise increases immune function, it is unclear whether exercise exacerbates or alleviates allergy states. No clear evidence exists of increased allergy prevalence in sedentary versus active people. Clearly allergic states can impede physical performance and activity through nasal obstruction, airway obstruction, rash, fatigue, headache, and even anaphylaxis. For convenience, the allergic condition is divided into seasonal allergic rhinitis and physical allergies. As discussed in chapter 1, physical allergies include a set of rare conditions brought on by exercise, including, but not limited to, cholinergic urticaria, cold urticaria, heat urticaria, solar urticaria, dermatographism, aquagenic urticaria, and exercise-induced anaphylaxis. Careful attention to symptoms, proper exercise planning, and adherence to an appropriate medical regimen will allow you to safely exercise if you have any of the aforementioned conditions.

Components of an Aerobic Exercise Program

An aerobic exercise program has several components: mode of exercise, intensity of exercise, duration of exercise, frequency of exercise, and progression of physical activity. For the purpose of this chapter, let's assume the mode of exercise to be walking, jogging or running, cycling, or swimming. Other modes of aerobic exercise will be discussed in later chapters. The following text will describe components of an aerobic exercise program tailored to individuals with asthma, EIA, seasonal allergies, and physical allergies. These components must be at a level to overload the normal function of the heart and lungs in order to produce an adaptive response, or training effect. Daily living tasks (bathing, cooking, cleaning, and walking from room to room) will place a load on your heart and lungs, but the components of these tasks do not meet the minimum levels to produce an adaptive response. It is paramount that you determine appropriate levels of intensity, duration, and frequency of your aerobic exercise program to gain a training effect, but more important, to avoid stressing your body too much.

Modes of Aerobic Exercise

Walking

Jogging

Running

Cycling

Swimming

Cross-country skiing

Hiking

Snowshoeing

Rowing

Jumping rope

Dancing

Intensity

Our bodies can run on different types of fuel. Instead of leaded or unleaded fuel, our bodies (muscles and other cells) run on aerobic and anaerobic metabolism. Aerobic metabolism produces energy without the waste products associated with anaerobic metabolism. The body needs oxygen to run aerobically. If the heart and lungs cannot provide that oxygen in a timely manner, the body meets its energy need through anaerobic metabolism. Anaerobic metabolism produces lactic acid. The body cannot function with a large excess of lactic acid.

Swimming is a good example of how intensity relates to aerobic exercise performance. A 50- or 100-meter swimmer is able to swim short distances at high speed. A 5,000-meter swimmer can swim long distances and maintain a relatively slower speed. If these two swimmers were to face each other in a 1,000-meter race, the sprinter would not be able to maintain intensity (speed and power) for long and would eventually slow the swim pace. The distance swimmer would adapt by increasing intensity to increase the swim pace.

When you start to exercise, your body will determine the power needed to perform your chosen activity and its intensity. The nervous system will first recruit small aerobic muscle groups and then large mixed aerobic and anaerobic muscle groups. The more intense the exercise, the more anaerobic muscle groups will be recruited in addition to the smaller aerobic muscle groups. To that end, as exercise intensity increases oxygen must be delivered quickly. The lungs will increase ventilation rate and lung volume. The heart will increase rate and volume of blood pumped for each beat. The vascular system will increase blood volume and red blood cells. If exercise intensity exceeds the body's oxygen delivery capacity, the body will switch to anaerobic metabolism and produce lactic acid that the body will clear. This point is your $\dot{V}O_2max$. The heart rate is the most readily measured sign directly related to $\dot{V}O_2max$. (For a review, refer to the discussion on $\dot{V}O_2max$ in chapter 2.)

The rhythmic and repetitive nature of aerobic exercise will train the nervous system to recruit aerobic muscle groups. The muscles will adapt by increasing size of aerobic muscle groups and number of aerobic muscle units. The heart and lungs will adapt as mentioned previously. These adaptations will increase your $\dot{V}O_2max$ about 15 to 25 percent over time. If you start at too high an intensity, the body will convert to anaerobic metabolism and create a different training effect. You probably can never start too low, but if the intensity is below the threshold to stimulate adaptation, it will take longer to reap the benefits of exercise.

All modes of aerobic exercise may be performed at differing intensities, and each person will experience differing intensities for the same activity. The beginning intensity for each aerobic exercise program is individually based. Before determining your level of exercise intensity, consider the factors mentioned in the following sidebar. We focus on asthma, EIA, and allergies later in this chapter. Exercise intensity is directly related to $\dot{V}O_2$max, and $\dot{V}O_2$max is linearly related to heart rate. To determine intensity you need to know resting and maximal heart rate. The maximal heart rate is commonly estimated by subtracting one's age from the number 220. Thus, the closer your heart rate is to the maximal heart rate, the closer you are to maximum intensity, or $\dot{V}O_2$max. If the resting heart rate is abnormally high or low, this method may not be ideal. The heart rate reserve method discussed next is an alternative estimate that accounts for resting heart rate.

Factors to Consider When Determining Intensity

The following conditions, depending on their status, may limit your starting exercise intensity and your goal intensity. Be honest with yourself. If you over- or underestimate your ability, you will be less likely to stick to your program and reap the benefits.

▸ Fitness level at present time

▸ Cardiovascular health

▸ Pulmonary health

▸ Orthopedic conditions

▸ Goal of exercise program

▸ Goal of individual starting the exercise program

▸ Individual preferences for exercise

ACSM (2005) suggests that individuals exercise in a range of maximal heart rate and heart rate reserve. The older guidelines suggest a range of 55 to 90 percent of maximal heart rate, and newer guidelines advocate 50 to 85 percent of heart rate reserve. Exercising in this range stimulates the body to adapt and consequently improve function. However, for very sedentary individuals or individuals with comorbid conditions, an initial intensity of 40 to 50 percent may provide cardiovascular and respiratory benefits (ACSM 2005). The range serves to start higher-risk individuals at the lower end range. So, you should start at the low end range and use the heart rate reserve method unless you have consulted a physician regarding exercise prescription. You can determine heart rate reserve (or target heart rate, as it will be referred to from here on) using the Karvonen formula shown in chapter 2 (page 21). This formula adjusts for resting heart rates that lie outside the normal limits, an important consideration, because each individual is physiologically different and may be on medications that change resting heart rate.

Establishing Individual Exercise Intensity

To determine your exercise intensity range, you must be able to calculate your resting heart rate. A simple method involves palpating your radial artery: Place the tips of your right index finger and middle finger just below the base of your left thumb. Apply gentle pressure with your fingertips. Once you feel the pulse, count the number of pulsations over a 10-second period. Then multiply that number by 6 to determine your resting heart rate (number of heart beats in 1 minute). You should check your resting heart rate upon waking or after 5 minutes of rest during the day. Do not use your thumb to feel for your pulse, because it has a pulse of its own, which may make it difficult to accurately assess your resting heart rate.

Once you know your resting heart rate, you should figure your target heart rate range using the Karvonen formula. For example, assuming you want to exercise within 50 to 85 percent of your maximal intensity, you would multiply .5 and .85 by your maximum heart rate to get an acceptable training heart rate range. It is very difficult to achieve and sustain an exact heart rate. You can determine target heart rate ranges by 10-second heart rate counts, give or take a beat for each 10-second interval (table 3.1). You should try to exercise within this target heart rate range.

Table 3.1   Estimated Heart Rates by 10-Second Count

10-second count	Beats per minute	10-second count	Beats per minute
10 beats	60	18 beats	108
11 beats	66	19 beats	114
12 beats	72	20 beats	120
13 beats	78	21 beats	126
14 beats	84	22 beats	132
15 beats	90	23 beats	138
16 beats	96	24 beats	144
17 beats	102	25 beats	150

Reprinted, by permission, from A.L. Millar, 2003, *Action plan for arthritis* (Champaign, IL: Human Kinetics), 53.

The rating of perceived exertion (RPE) method is for those who have difficulty measuring heart rate, want a simpler measurement of intensity, or have an altered physiologic heart rate response (i.e., from medication). RPE should be considered adjunctive to other methods of determining intensity because it does not consistently reflect intensity of varying modes of aerobic exercise or intensity of a graded exercise session. The RPE is a useful tool to estimate intensity but should not replace the heart rate reserve and target heart rate range as the absolute indicator of intensity. You may use the RPE as a subjective measurement to confirm your estimated target ranges calculated by the Karvonen formula. RPE measures intensity on the Borg scale (see figure 3.1).

6	No exertion at all
7	Extremely light
8	
9	Very light
10	
11	Light
12	
13	Somewhat hard
14	
15	Hard (heavy)
16	
17	Very hard
18	
19	Extremely hard
20	Maximal exertion

Figure 3.1 Borg's RPE scale.

Reprinted, by permission, from G. Borg, 1998, *Borg's Perceived Exertion and Pain Scales* (Champaign, IL: Human Kinetics), 47.

Setting Your Own Intensity

Several factors should be considered when setting your initial target heart rate range and intensity. Many of you may feel age and sex may determine on which end of the intensity range you will begin, but you shouldn't concern yourself with these factors. They play very little role in determining exercise intensity. For instance, a sedentary, young man would likely benefit from starting at the lower end of his target heart rate, but this level would less likely benefit an older, already fit and active woman. The key is to stick to your exercise program. A common mistake is to start off too intense and quit your beneficial aerobic exercise program because of frustration or injury. Remember, you only need to stress the body enough to stimulate beneficial physiologic adaptive changes. You may achieve similar physiologic benefits for lower-intensity, longer-duration exercise programs as with higher-intensity, shorter-duration exercise programs. A higher incidence of musculoskeletal and cardiovascular injury is associated with higher-intensity exercise programs. This risk is accentuated when a very sedentary individual immediately exercises at the high end percentage of target heart rate. Always err on the side of caution: Start low and go slow. You can evaluate your current level of activity by determining whether you are sedentary, moderately active, or active. Sedentary individuals engage in mild activity about 2 days a week. Moderately active individuals engage in moderate activity about 2 or 3 days a week. Active individuals engage in vigorous activity about 3 to 5 days a week (see table 3.2). Sedentary, moderately active, and active individuals should begin an aerobic exercise program with intensities of 55 to 65, 65 to 75, and 75 to 85 percent of target heart rate, respectively. Again, this guideline can be adjusted based on individual differences.

Table 3.2   Intensity of Leisure Activities

Mild-intensity activity	Moderate-intensity activity	High-intensity activity
Bowling	Hiking (flat)	Running/jogging
Fishing	Cycling (pleasure)	Cycling 10 mph
Golf (cart)	Golfing (walking)	Racquetball
Shuffleboard	Swimming	Cross-country skiing
Slow walking	Skating (leisure)	Backpacking

When you are exercising at an intensity of 55 to 65 percent of your target heart rate, you should be able to hold a conversation. As you increase your intensity to 65 to 75 percent, you may only be able to say a sentence or two without difficult. The closer you get to your target heart rate range, the more difficult conversation will be; maybe a short phrase will be all you can muster. Muscle soreness, breathlessness, and cramping are signs that you are near your maximal fatigue level. These symptoms occur when your body cannot supply enough oxygen to the working muscles and lactic acid waste products start to build. So, exercising beyond this point may increase the risk of injury.

As mentioned previously, consult your physician or health care provider before exercising if you have any ongoing medical conditions or take any medications. Asthma, EIA, allergic rhinitis, and physical allergies are no exception to this rule. These conditions require additional considerations before setting your initial exercise intensity. You need to find out whether your asthma is under control. You should take a peak flow measurement, and if it is within 80 percent of your best or ideal peak flow with no wheezing, coughing, chest discomfort, or difficulty breathing, you're ready for exercise. Peak flow readings less than 80 percent, as well as the symptoms stated earlier, indicate your asthma is not under adequate control (see tables 3.3 and 3.4). In this case, you should perform a warm-up of slightly lower intensity (about 10 to 15 percent lower) than the exercise session. This low-intensity warm-up can produce 45 to 60 minutes of exercise time refractory to bronchospasm or wheezing. You should always premedicate

Table 3.3   Predicted Average Peak Expiratory Flow for Men

Age (years)	Height (inches)				
	60	65	70	75	80
20	554	602	649	693	740
25	543	590	636	679	725
30	532	577	622	664	710
35	521	565	609	651	695
40	509	552	596	636	680
45	498	540	583	622	665
50	486	527	569	607	649
55	475	515	556	593	634
60	463	502	542	578	618
65	452	490	529	564	603
70	440	477	515	550	587

Peak flow values in liters per minute.
From C.G. Leiner, et al., 1963, "Expiratory peak flow rates," *American Review of Respiratory Disease,* vol. 88, p. 644. Official Journal of the American Thoratic Society.

Table 3.4   Predicted Average Peak Expiratory Flow for Women

Age (years)	Height (inches)				
	55	60	65	70	75
20	390	423	460	496	529
25	385	418	454	490	523
30	380	413	448	483	516
35	375	408	442	476	509
40	370	402	436	470	502
45	365	397	430	464	495
50	360	391	424	457	488
55	355	386	418	451	482
60	350	380	412	445	475
65	345	375	406	439	468
70	340	369	400	432	461

Peak flow values in liters per minute.
From C.G. Leiner, et al., 1963, "Expiratory peak flow rates," *American Review of Respiratory Disease,* vol. 88, p. 644. Official Journal of the American Thoratic Society.

with two puffs of your rescue inhaler before your warm-up and take your asthma maintenance medications on a regular basis. If you experience coughing, wheezing, excessive shortness of breath, or chest discomfort, your intensity level is likely too high. You should stop, administer two puffs of your rescue inhaler, and check your peak flow. Further discussion regarding preparation for exercise with asthma and EIA will be discussed later in this chapter.

Allergic rhinitis or hay fever should not prevent you from exercising. However, uncontrolled allergies may cause sinus and upper airway congestion, fatigue, and limited ability to exercise at higher intensities. Further, certain allergic reactions may trigger more serious physical allergies (discussed later in this chapter). Following a specific medication schedule and carefully choosing the exercise environment should minimize problems from allergic rhinitis and physical allergies (hives, rashes, and other systemic symptoms).

Duration

Just as your initial exercise intensity should be based on your current activity level, you should treat your initial duration of exercise sessions similarly. Also, pay particular attention to the severity of your asthma and allergies. ACSM's current recommendation for initial duration of exercise is 20 to 60 minutes of continuous or intermittent aerobic activity accumulated throughout the day (ACSM 2005). This time does not include adequate warm-up and cool-down periods. The duration of an exercise session will, in concert with intensity, determine the amount of work produced to achieve all the health benefits stated previously. If possible, perform continuous aerobic activity for maximal benefits. However, don't be frustrated if you can only exercise in short durations. Similar benefits may be achieved with frequent, short bouts of exercise as longer, less frequent bouts of exercise. Shorter bouts of intermittent activity throughout the day may be a better and safer alternative to 20 to 60 minutes of continuous activity. If you try to exercise too long, too soon, your risk of injury will increase and you probably will not stay with your exercise program.

Pay attention to your body. Coughing, wheezing, breathlessness, and chest discomfort are all signs you're exercising too long or too hard. This is a good time to stop, check your peak flow, use your rescue inhaler, and adjust your exercise duration. Exercising shorter durations outdoors during different allergy seasons may minimize allergy or asthma symptoms. To augment shortened outdoor exercise durations you may consider joining an indoor gym or purchasing exercise equipment during high pollen count seasons. Try adding indoor swimming to augment cumulative exercise duration, along with already shortened bouts of outdoor exercise. The pool provides a warmer, moist environment that is easier on asthma and allergies. The exception would be chlorine sensitivity or a rare physical allergy, aquagenic urticaria.

The best exercise program is the one that works for you, the one that you will continue to follow. We are living in a fast-paced society and feel overwhelmed much of the time, but exercise should be a part of a healthy lifestyle no matter how busy we have become. I'm sure you want to jump right in at the suggested ideal intensity and duration; but your physical condition, medical conditions, and activity level may not allow it. Modify your duration of exercise to ensure your safety and compliance with your program. The ideal exercise duration is 20 to 60 minutes of continuous, rhythmic, and repetitive movement at a minimal threshold of intensity. If your schedule does not allow for the ideal, feel free to combine short bouts of exercise to achieve the desired cumulative duration of aerobic activity. This is your exercise program, you own it, and only you can determine what is feasible for you to achieve.

Frequency

ACSM recommends an average of 3 to 5 aerobic exercise sessions a week to achieve and maintain cardiovascular, respiratory, musculoskeletal, metabolic, and weight-loss benefits from your exercise program. As with the other essential components of exercise, the frequency of sessions should be tailored to the individual. Many national health authorities recommend you be active all days of the week, but it does not mean you have to exercise every day of the week. Assuming you are exercising within 60 to 85 percent of your target heart rate, you may only need to exercise 3 sessions a week. It is natural to think a higher frequency may provide further health benefits, but if your 3 sessions a week are set at the proper intensity and duration, ample evidence exists to the contrary. The ACSM 2005 guidelines note that intense aerobic exercise sessions 3 times a week will maintain your current level of cardiovascular and respiratory fitness (ACSM 2005). Hickson et al. (1985) demonstrated that reductions in intensity of training resulted in loss of training effect over duration and frequency. You should consider exercising 5 sessions a week if your activity level and physical condition prohibit adequate intensity and duration of exercise. Further, you may want to engage in 1 or 2 short sessions of low-level aerobic activity each day to gain a cumulative effect. Ample evidence supports that only minimal gains exist in health benefits from more frequent exercise sessions. It is clear that you stand a much higher chance of sustaining overuse injuries when exercising more than 5 sessions of 20 to 60 minutes of aerobic exercise each week. Consequently, these injuries will likely prevent you from enjoying and complying with your new exercise program.

You may modify frequency of certain aerobic activities to accommodate asthma, EIA, allergic rhinitis, and physical allergies. Reducing the frequency of outdoor exercise and increasing the frequency of indoor exercise may reduce exposure to allergens and unfavorable weather conditions that may exacerbate your asthma or other allergic conditions. Reduced allergen exposure can occur through engaging in alternative indoor activities, including spinning, swimming, dancing, circuit training, and jumping rope, and using equipment such as the treadmill, elliptical machine, or rowing machine. Again, it is your exercise program and you should modify the program within specific guidelines where you see fit.

Elements of the Exercise Session

Each exercise session, much like an exercise program, has several key elements that must be present to consider a session complete. The essential components are warm-up, endurance phase, and cool-down. You can incorporate an elective recreational activity, such as a game, into the endurance phase. Each of these components is dependent on the other to endure a safe and enjoyable exercise session.

Warm-Up Phase

The warm-up is an essential transition for your body from a resting state to exercise. The warm-up facilitates dynamic stretching of muscles, increases blood flow to muscles, and raises the metabolic rate to the required level for aerobic training. Scientific investigation has shown 10 to 15 minutes of warm-up significantly reduces postexercise bronchospasm. Studies have also shown that a proper warm-up will diminish postexercise airway restriction, a refractory period to asthma attacks (Reiff et al. 1989; McKenzie, McLuckie, and Stirling 1994; and Fitch, Morton, and Blanksby 1976). The refractory period was defined as a 2-hour time period following low-intensity aerobic activity not susceptible to further bronchospasm. Your warm-up should consist of 5 minutes of low-intensity, calisthenic-type exercises with a progression to 5 to 10 minutes of a lower-intensity version of the endurance phase mode of exercise (see table 3.5). For example, if you are going to run for 20 minutes, your warm-up should probably include 5 to 10 minutes of lower-intensity jogging. A continuous low-intensity warm-up is preferred over a warm-up session with varying intensities.

The warm-up is particularly paramount in asthma, EIA, and other allergic conditions. The low-intensity warm-up allows the lungs to adapt to the new environment and reduces the chances of wheezing and inflammation

Table 3.5 *Warm-Up and Cool-Down Guidelines*

Warm-up	Cool-down
5 min of calisthenics	5-10 min at 50% intensity
5-10 min at 50% intensity	Stretching
Stretching	Hydration and recovery nutrition

in the lungs. A warm-up may delay bronchospasm for 45 to 60 minutes, allowing for ample time to exercise safely. The warm-up is an excellent time to check your peak flow, determine whether it is at least 80 percent of your normal peak flow, and premedicate with two puffs of your rescue inhaler. Stretching is a key component to any warm-up session. I recommend stretching after your warm-up to reduce the chance of joint injury and improve proprioception.

Endurance Phase

The meat of your exercise session is the endurance phase. This 20- to 60-minute phase of continuous or intermittent aerobic activity provides the stimulus for improving fitness. The amount of stimulus depends heavily on intensity and duration of aerobic exercise. As stated before, you may adjust your intensity and duration to fit your individual needs. Augmenting a mode of aerobic exercise with a recreational sport during the endurance phase will provide similar fitness benefits. Ideally you should choose a sport that involves repetitive, rhythmic, and dynamic use of large muscle groups. The same principle of intensity and duration applies to recreational games. Basketball, racquetball, handball, and tennis are likely to be more intense than golf or bowling. If you add a recreational sport to your endurance phase, make sure you account for environmental exposure (pollen count, air pollution, humidity level, and temperature) because certain games may occur in conditions that can exacerbate asthma and allergies. Also, you may modify the rules of the game to allow for varying intensity of exercise. You may modify the playing field size to facilitate more or less continuous movement throughout the game and thus more or less aerobic intensity. Changing the height of a basket or net may make the game more difficult and facilitate more continuous aerobic activity and intensity. Employing a player rotation schedule will serve to equalize all the participants' aerobic activity level. For example, the ACSM guidelines (2005) suggest a volleyball match allowing for one bounce of the ball to promote continuous play. This modification will likely increase intensity and allow the participants to enjoy their exercise session. Be creative; you want to look forward to your exercise session.

Cool-Down Phase

The cool-down phase is your body's transition from an intense, metabolically active state to a resting, less active state. You should perform a similar, but less intense, activity to allow your heart rate, blood pressure, and respiratory rate to return to normal while maintaining adequate blood flow to vital structures. Abrupt cessation of exercise without a cool-down period decreases blood return to the heart. This reaction may cause fainting, dizziness, poor oxygenation of blood, and accumulation of metabolic waste products. The cool-down phase allows the body an easier transition from natural, exercise-induced, elevations of hormones. For instance, the body dilates blood vessels to increase blood flow to the muscles. If exercise is abruptly halted, the blood is still shunted to the muscle and may produce dizziness or fainting. A cool-down allows the body to slowly adjust back to the resting state, avoiding such complications. The cool-down phase should last about 5 to 15 minutes depending on the length of the endurance phase. You should cool down at 50 percent of your endurance phase intensity. The cool-down is an excellent opportunity to work on flexibility. Specific flexibility exercises are beyond the scope of this chapter but will be touched upon briefly in relation to specific modes of exercise. You can also include some strength training in your cool-down. You should not only strengthen the extremities but also the trunk muscles to prevent injury and improve performance. Stretching and strengthening exercises that mimic the functional movement of your chosen mode of exercise are the most beneficial. Physical therapists and certified athletic trainers are excellent sources for stretching and strengthening routines.

The cool-down phase is also a good opportunity to determine whether you can progress to a higher intensity, longer duration, or increased frequency. Monitor your symptoms. Any postexercise coughing, wheezing, chest discomfort, or breathlessness are indications you may need to stay at this level or reduce your level for the next exercise session. You should monitor your peak flow at the end of your cool-down and always have your rescue inhaler handy. A peak flow of 60 to 80 percent average peak, especially with symptoms, necessitates use of your rescue inhaler. If you exercise outside and go inside, or vice versa, the cool-down will bring your body back to a normal physiologic state before placing the stress of a different environment on your body, especially your lungs and allergies. For instance, immediately going from a warm, climate-controlled gym to a dry, cold winter environment certainly may trigger bronchospasm. Further, moving from an indoor exercise facility to the outdoors without performing a proper cool-down during a high-pollen-count day could exacerbate your asthma and allergies more than normal. A good rule of thumb is to warm up, exercise, and cool down in the same environment.

Sample Cardiovascular Exercise Programs

Familiarity with the essential components of an exercise program and of an exercise session is paramount to analyzing your current exercise regimen. Now, the goal of this chapter is to help you apply these principles to a new mode of exercise or modify and augment your existing exercise program. As stated before, these guidelines are just that; they are not intended to replace the expertise of your health care professional. Aerobic exercise involves rhythmic, repetitive movements of large muscle groups. The most popular and easiest modes of aerobic exercise to perform are walking, jogging or running, cycling, and swimming. This section outlines beginning to advanced exercise programs for each of these activities and discusses how they relate to asthma, allergic rhinitis, and physical allergies.

Walking

Walking is an excellent mode of aerobic exercise. It will stimulate your body to produce adaptive changes beneficial to your everyday function. Walking will increase your pulmonary capacity to tolerate increasing levels of activities and decrease your risk of cardiovascular disease, among other benefits. By maintaining a walking program you will experience less coughing, wheezing, breathlessness, and chest discomfort with activity. You will still have asthma and allergies, but your activity tolerance should improve. Maybe you would like to play a tennis match or walk nine holes instead of taking a cart. Even with asthma and allergies, a proper walking program may get you the endurance you need. Allergic rhinitis and EIA should not prevent you from reaping the benefits of a walking program. Allergy avoidance and proper medications should allow you to participate.

Careful preparation before exercise will minimize complications and increase your enjoyment of the walking program. First, determine whether you are fit enough to start a walking program. Generally, if you are under 40 years old without medical problems, you probably can safely start a walking program. It is always a good idea to visit your personal physician before beginning an exercise program, but if you are over 40 and have any medical problems, you are strongly encouraged to schedule a visit. If you have moderate to severe asthma or your peak flow is consistently 60 to 80 percent of your predicted level, you should still be able to walk after consulting your physician. Your physician may recommend pulmonary function tests to determine the severity of your asthma and consequently your fitness for a walking program.

Equipment, Medication, and Environment

Choosing the right equipment for your walking program is important. Remember, you are the main factor in starting and maintaining a successful walking program. Expensive or high-tech equipment is unlikely to improve your performance. A less expensive shoe may be more ideally suited to your feet than an expensive, popular walking shoe. I recommend buying walking shoes from an athletic store specializing in running or walking shoes. Each person has unique feet; one type of shoe may be a good choice for your friend, but the same shoe may not be ideal for you. If you have flat feet or a flexible arch, you will likely benefit from a stiffer support shoe. If you have high-arched or rigid feet, you will likely benefit from a shoe designed for cushion or comfort. Wear clothing made from synthetic fibers to facilitate sweat evaporation and efficiently cool your body. Ideally your clothing should be light and loose to allow full range of motion. Use some type of mouth covering for exercising in a cold, dry, polluted, or high-pollen-count environment. A simple scarf or surgical mask will help increase the air temperature and reduce allergen exposure. Make sure you have pockets to carry your rescue inhaler, peak flow meter, or other medications—the most essential equipment for your walking program. Backpacks or waist packs are useful for carrying these items, too. Staying hydrated is very important; always have water readily available to maintain hydration. A pedometer may be a useful tool for monitoring your exercise session by quantifying the actual number of strides taken and distance traveled. To avoid accidents while exercising on a treadmill, always choose a treadmill with an emergency stop button, and be familiar with how to safely start and stop the treadmill. Sunscreen is always a good idea when exercising outdoors, and it is particularly important for solar urticaria. Long-sleeved shirts, jackets, caps, and long pants may be required for warmth or, in the case of solar urticaria, sun protection. You may minimize symptoms of cold urticaria by dressing properly for walking in the cold weather. In short, choose your equipment with an emphasis on function, not fashion.

Hydration Guidelines

▸ Drink water to thirst throughout the day.

▸ Drink 8 to 16 ounces of water 1 hour before exercise.

▸ Drink to thirst, about 12 to 24 ounces for each hour of exercise.

▸ When exercising longer than 60 minutes, use an electrolyte drink.

▸ Replenish your body with water or electrolyte drink after exercise.

Choose your exercise environment carefully. You can perform a walking program indoors on a treadmill, in a mall, or on an indoor track. You may prefer to walk outdoors. Pay close attention to temperature, humidity, and pollen counts. In general, higher temperatures, higher humidity, and lower pollen counts are better for asthma, EIA, and allergic rhinitis. However, exercising in hot, humid weather will increase your risk of dehydration, heat illness, and other complications. Exercising in moderate heat index and low pollen counts is ideal if you choose to exercise outdoors. The heat index is directly proportional to the level of heat and humidity. Conversely, walking on a treadmill in your basement may seem ideal, with lower temperatures and increased humidity. However, basements often have lots of mold and other allergens that may facilitate asthma and allergy attacks. Although pollen counts are lower in winter, the air is usually cold and dry, not an optimal environment to start walking with a history of asthma or EIA. Also, in an area with high air pollution exercising indoors may be beneficial. If you choose to walk in a suboptimal environment, pay careful attention to your local weather report and reduce your intensity or duration of exercise in unfavorable conditions.

Physical allergies are unique conditions that can be minimized. You can reduce symptoms of solar urticaria by exercising behind window glass, wearing appropriate clothing, and using sunscreen. You may minimize symptoms of cold urticaria by exercising indoors or wearing appropriate layers of clothing when outdoors. As discussed in chapter 2, if you have exercise-induced anaphylaxis, a rare and possibly fatal condition, exercise only with a partner or in a public place. Your partner should know how to administer medication by injection, and the place you choose to exercise should be prepared if anaphylaxis occurs.

Walking Programs

Each person has different levels of fitness when starting a walking program. Individuals may adjust the intensity, duration, or frequency to maximally benefit from their program. Tables 3.6, 3.7, and 3.8 provide guidelines of beginning, intermediate, and advanced walking programs for poorly fit, moderately fit, and very fit individuals, respectively. Each program consists of a conditioning stage, improvement stage, and maintenance stage. Each stage comprises approximately 4 weeks of exercise. The rate at which you progress depends on your exercise capacity, asthma control, EIA control, and tolerance to the level of training. When you reach the maintenance stage and continue to exercise at this level at a tolerable rating of perceived exertion without coughing, wheezing, chest discomfort, or breathlessness, you are ready to graduate. Ideally you will have peak flow values consistently greater than 80 percent of your personal best and decreased use of your rescue inhaler before progressing to another program level. Note that each progression incorporates change in only one component—intensity, duration, or frequency. ACSM does not recommend increasing frequency or duration simultaneously (ACSM 2005). Any time you experience asthma symptoms or a reduced peak flow during exercise, stop and use your rescue inhaler. It is best not to exercise that day, and when you do exercise again, reduce your intensity, duration, or frequency to the previous level for one week before you consider progression.

These guidelines are not meant to be specific for every individual. Your personal physician, physical therapist, or athletic trainer is the best source of information. Your fitness level or medical condition may not allow you to start at 40 to 50 percent of your target heart rate. I recommend using the RPE while monitoring your heart rate to gradually condition yourself to the ACSM recommended starting intensity. Consult your physician to ensure your asthma, allergies, or EIA are adequately treated to allow you to exercise. You may find that your fitness level is adequate but your medical condition was inhibiting you from starting at the recommended intensity. Your initial duration should be 15 to 20 minutes. As mentioned earlier, although continuous exercise is preferred, you may perform two sessions totaling 20 minutes if your fitness level requires this modification. The initial frequency of exercise should be 3 sessions a week. Always include

Table 3.6 Initial Walking Program

Initial phase		Improvement phase		Maintenance phase	
Week	Exercise components	Weeks	Exercise components	Week(s)	Exercise components
1	I: 40% THR D: 5-7 min 3/day F: 3/week	7-9	I: 45-50% THR D: 25-30 min/day F: 4-5/week		
2	I: 40% THR D: 10 min 2/day F: 3/week	10-12	I: 45-50% THR D: 30 min/day F: 5/week		
3	I: 40-45% THR D: 10 min 2/day F: 3-4/week	13-15	I: 50% THR D: 30 min/day F: 5/week		
4	I: 40-45% THR D: 12-15 min 2/day F: 3-4/week	16-18	I: 50% THR D: 30-35 min/day F: 5/week		
5	I: 45% THR D: 12-15 min 2/day F: 4/week	19-21	I: 50-55% THR D: 30-35 min/day F: 5-7/week		
6	I: 45% THR D: 25 min 1/day F: 4/week	22-24	I: 50-55% THR D: 35 min/day F: 5-7/week	25+	I: 55% THR D: 35 min/day F: 5-7/week C: Hills or flat

I = intensity; D = duration; F = frequency; C = course; THR = target heart rate
Always exercise on alternate days when possible.

Table 3.7   Intermediate Walking Program

Initial phase		Improvement phase		Maintenance phase	
Week	Exercise components	Weeks	Exercise components	Week(s)	Exercise components
1	I: 50% THR D: 10 min 3/day F: 5/week	7-9	I: 55-60% THR D: 35 min/day F: 5/week		
2	I: 50% THR D: 15 min 2/day F: 5/week	10-12	I: 55-60% THR D: 40 min/day F: 5/week		
3	I: 50-55% THR D: 15 min 2/day F: 5/week	13-15	I: 60% THR D: 40 min/day F: 5/week		
4	I: 50-55% THR D: 30 min/day F: 5/week	16-18	I: 60% THR D: 40 min/day F: 5-7/week		
5	I: 55% THR D: 30 min/day F: 5/week	19-21	I: 60-65% THR D: 40 min/day F: 5-7/week		
6	I: 55% THR D: 35 min/day F: 5/week	22-24	I: 60-65% THR D: 45 min/day F: 5-7/week	25+	I: 65% THR D: 45 min/day F: 5-7/week C: Hills or flat

I = intensity; D = duration; F = frequency; C = course; THR = target heart rate
Always exercise on alternate days when possible.

Table 3.8   Advanced Walking Program

Day	Initial phase — Week 1 exercise components	Improvement phase — Week 2 exercise components	Improvement phase — Week 3 exercise components	Maintenance phase — Week 4 exercise components	Maintenance phase — Week 5 + exercise components
Monday	I: 60-65% THR D: 30 min C: Flat	I: 65-70% THR D: 35 min C: Flat	I: 70-75% THR D: 40 min C: Flat	I: 75% THR D: 40 min C: Hills or elevate treadmill	I: 70-85% THR D: 40-60 min C: Hills or flat
Tuesday	I: 60-65% THR D: 35 min C: Flat	I: 65-70% THR D: 35 min C: Flat	I: 70-75% THR D: 40 minutes C: Flat	I: 75% THR D: 45 min C: Hills or elevated treadmill	I: 70-85% THR D: 40-60 min C: Hills or flat
Wednesday	I: 65% THR D: 40 min C: Flat	I: 70% THR D: 40 min C: Flat	I: 75% THR D: 45 min C: Flat	I: 75-80% THR D: 45 min C: Flat	I: 70-85% THR D: 40-60 min C: Hills of flat
Thursday	I: 65% THR D: 40 min C: Hills or elevated treadmill	I: 70% THR D: 45 min C: Hills or elevated treadmill	I: 75% THR D: 45 min C: Hills or elevated treadmill	I: 75-80% THR D: 50 min C: Flat	I: 70-85% THR D: 40-60 min C: Hills or flat
Friday	Rest or other mode of aerobic exercise	Rest or other mode of aerobic exercise	Rest or other mode of aerobic exercise	Rest or other mode of aerobic exercise	Rest or other mode of aerobic exercise
Saturday	I: 70% THR D: 40 min C: Flat	I: 75% THR D: 45 min C: Flat	I: 80% THR D: 50 min C: Flat	I: 80% THR D: 50 min C: Hills or elevated treadmill	I: 70-85% THR D: 40-60 min C: Hills or flat
Sunday	I: 55% THR D: 45 min C: Flat	I: 55% THR D: 50 min C: Flat	I: 55% THR D: 55 min C: Flat	I: 55% THR D: 60 min C: Flat	I: 55% THR D: 60 min C: Flat

I = intensity; D = duration; F = frequency; C = course; THR = target heart rate
Always exercise on alternate days if possible, and always incorporate a rest day.

an adequate warm-up and cool-down. The lighter intensity, duration, and frequency are designed to limit complications from asthma and allergy to ensure enjoyment of and compliance to your exercise program. Doing too much, too soon certainly will place you at higher risk for an asthma attack and hinder your progress or worse.

Some of you may already be moderately active and find the initial program too easy. If you desire longer, more intense exercise sessions and plan to start a higher-level program, visit your health care provider to accurately determine your fitness level. For example, you may consider obtaining pulmonary function tests to determine the severity of your asthma. The initial intensity is set at 50 to 55 percent of target heart rate and gradually rises each month for 3 months. The duration ranges from 30 to 40 minutes. The frequency is five to seven sessions a week. Do not be overzealous when increasing the intensity or duration. You may find you are fitter than you thought, but you should still slowly increase your intensity or duration to avoid complications. It is best to increase the duration before intensity to reduce complication from asthma and EIA.

Some very fit individuals may want to add walking to their current exercise program. Table 3.9 on page 67 provides a guideline for such a program. Generally this program includes higher intensity and somewhat higher durations with similar frequency of exercise sessions. Fit individuals may be adding a walking program to increase variety of exercise. Try varying your walking routine to prevent boredom. Changing walking courses, treadmill grades, and exercise environment may help. Walking with a partner or group may be more enjoyable. The more you enjoy walking, the more you are likely to adhere to the program. Incorporating a rest day or alternative exercise day will reduce the risk of overuse injuries and increase enjoyment.

Adequate warm-up and cool-down sessions are also essential to gain maximal benefit from your walking program and prevent injury. Be conservative with exercise progression; too much, too soon may increase risk of injuries and complications from asthma and EIA. Lastly, always carry your rescue inhaler, and enjoy your walking program.

Running and Jogging

Running and jogging are excellent choices for aerobic exercise. I view jogging and running as a continuum of activity. Both exercises use large muscle groups (extremity and trunk) in repetitive, rhythmic motion. Both modes of exercise are weight-bearing activities. The differences are the level of impact on your joints and load placed on your cardiovascular and pulmonary system. Running tends to be higher impact and performed at higher intensity. These exercises should produce a higher intensity session than a walking program. You should be able to easily complete a moderate- to high-level walking program before adding running or jogging. These activities are higher impact and may stimulate the body to higher ventilation rates, higher oxygen demand, and increased metabolic activity.

Your activity level should be in the moderate to high level before considering adding a running or jogging program. Start with a walking program, and gradually increase your walking speed until you can easily maintain a brisk walking pace before jogging or running. You probably can jog or run slowly enough to exercise at 40 to 50 percent of your target heart rate, but the higher impact of jogging or running may increase your risk of injury. If you are jogging or running at a very slow pace, consider changing to walking for similar cardiovascular gains with less risk of injury. You may have been a runner in the past. If you have not gained a lot of weight and have stayed moderately active, you may be able to begin jogging and gradually change into running. Excess weight can worsen asthma and EIA, and if your weight fluctuates, your exercise tolerance will follow. Approximately 50 percent of the training effect is lost after 1 or 2 months of sedentary behavior. If it has been more than 2 months since you consistently ran, start now with walking or jogging. The idea is to condition your heart and lungs during walking so that when energy demand increases with jogging or running, your body is efficient and doesn't require you to take rapid, shallow breaths to keep up with demand. Rapid, shallow or deep breathing exposes the lungs to allergens, decreases lung temperature and humidity, and facilitates airway restriction. Remember, running does not reduce the severity of asthma or EIA more than walking, but it provides higher-intensity training and increased conditioning. This in turn may allow you to tolerate higher levels of varying exercise modes.

Equipment, Medication, and Environment

I have been surprised by the process runners go through when choosing running shoes. Many runners are very dedicated and pay particular attention to detail. However, I find the majority of runners choose shoes based on brand, price, or aesthetics. Every individual's feet require varying amounts of support, cushion, or control. Pay close attention to the midsole of the shoe and the heel cup. Just as with walking, you may need more support or more cushion in the midsole and a rigid or softer heel cup for flat or high-arched feet, respectively. The shoe is very important for running because the impact to the body is greater. Change your shoes every 300 miles; the midsole loses its support and cushion, and a worn tread occurs long after the support or cushioning elements have left the shoe. Local shoe stores that specialize in running shoes are your best bet for finding an appropriate running shoe. Light, loose-fitting clothing with pockets is ideal. Use lighter clothing in warm weather and layers in cooler weather. Carry your rescue inhaler (or other medication), peak flow meter, and water if it is not available on the course. A surgical mask or scarf may be used in the cold, dry air or during high-pollen-count or high-pollution days if you are exercising outdoors. As stated previously, clothing choices, sunscreen application, and proper exercise environment can minimize physical allergies (solar and cold urticaria), allergic rhinitis, asthma, and EIA. Optimizing the environment for exercise is discussed in greater detail later in this book.

Running and Jogging Programs

Jogging and running are more physically demanding than walking. These activities require work from similar muscle groups but at a higher intensity. Your minute ventilation, how quickly and deeply you breathe, will increase to supply adequate oxygen to these working muscles. You should be able to comfortably walk at 60 percent of your target heart rate for 30 to 35 minutes before considering the initial program outlined in table 3.9. Also, your peak flow should be more than 80 percent of predicted and you should not experience coughing, wheezing, chest tightness, or breathlessness while walking 30 to 35 minutes at 60 percent of your target heart rate. The initial phase, weeks 1 through 4, will concentrate on increasing the duration of the exercise session with a moderate increase in intensity. The improvement phase, weeks 5 through 24, consists of equally increasing intensities and durations. When you reach the maintenance phase, you can really personalize your program to combat boredom or reach other individual goals. I have added changes in the course, hilly or flat, to vary the method of changing intensity and to facilitate use of different muscle groups. Anytime you experience persistent EIA or asthma symptoms, consider falling back one exercise block and do not advance to the next block. Take at least one day of rest, strength training, or cross-training. When you reach the maintenance phase I recommend incorporating a strength training program or biking or swimming twice a week to avoid overuse injuries.

Some of you may already be jogging or running a couple times a week along with other exercise. The advanced program offers higher-intensity training for people who are already fit. Peak flow measurements and asthma symptoms should be under good control before beginning this program. You should not be experiencing more than one or two episodes of EIA to start the advanced jogging or running program (table 3.10). The same principle applies to asthma symptoms. Jogging symptom free for 30 to 40 minutes at 65 to 70 percent of your target heart rate, twice a week is an indication you're ready for this program. The principals of progression are similar to those of the initial program but at higher intensities and longer durations. Try signing up for a community 5K or 10K race as a goal. It will keep your interest and give you more of a sense of accomplishment. Running clubs or running with a partner also should keep you motivated. Remember to take your medications, carry your rescue inhaler, keep yourself hydrated, work on flexibility, and incorporate strength training into your routine. Mostly, you should personalize your routine to maximize your enjoyment of running.

Table 3.9 Initial Jogging or Running Program

Initial phase				
	Week 1	**Week 2**	**Week 3**	**Week 4**
Exercise components	I: 65% THR D: 20-30 min jogging in intervals F: 5-7/week C: Flat	I: 65% THR D: 20-30 min jogging continuously F: 5-7/week C: Flat	I: 65-70% THR D: 20-30 min jogging continuously F: 5-7/week C: Flat or hills	I: 70% THR D: 30-40 min jogging continuously F: 5-7/week C: Flat
Monday	10 min 2/day	20 min	20 min hill course	30 min
Tuesday	12 min 2/day	25 min	25 min flat course	35 min
Wednesday	15 min 2/day	30 min	30 min flat course	40 min
Thursday	12 min 2/day	25 min	25 min hill course	30 min
Friday	Rest, strength, or other mode	Rest, strength, or other mode	Rest, strength, or other mode	Rest, strength, or other mode
Saturday	15 min 2/day	30 min	30 min hill course	40 min
Sunday	12 min 2/day	25 min	25 min flat course	35 min
Improvement phase				
	Weeks 5-9	**Weeks 10-14**	**Weeks 15-19**	**Weeks 20-24**
Exercise components	I: 70%-75% THR D: 30-40 min jogging continuously F: 5-7/week C: Flat	I: 70-75% THR D: 30-40 min jogging continuously F: 5-7/week C: Flat or hills	I: 75-80% THR D: 40-50 min jogging continuously F: 5-7/week C: Flat	I: 75-80% THR D: 40-50 min jogging continuously F: 5-7/week C: Flat or hills
Monday	30 min	30 min hill course	40 min	40 min hill course
Tuesday	35 min	35 min flat course	45 min	45 min flat course
Wednesday	40 min	40 min flat course	50 min	50 min flat course
Thursday	35 min	35 min hill course	45 min	45 min hill course
Friday	Rest, strength, or other mode	Rest, strength, or other mode	Rest, strength, or other mode	Rest, strength, or other mode
Saturday	40 min	40 min hill course	50 min	50 min hill course
Sunday	35 min	35 min flat course	45 min	45 min flat course
Maintenance phase				
	Weeks 25+			
Exercise components	I: 70-85% THR D: 40-60 min jogging continuously F: 3/week C: Flat or hills			
Monday-Sunday	Combine the above components to achieve 70-85% THR to maintain training effect.			

I = intensity; D = duration; F = frequency; C = course; THR = target heart rate
Always exercise on alternate days if possible, and always incorporate a rest day.

Table 3.10   Advanced Jogging or Running Program

	Initial phase			
	Week 1	**Week 2**	**Week 3**	**Week 4**
Exercise components	I: 70-75% THR D: 30-40 min jogging continuously F: 5-7/week C: Flat	I: 70-75% THR D: 30-40 min jogging continuously F: 5-7/week C: Flat or hills	I:70-75% THR D: 40-50 min jogging continuously F: 5-7/week C: Flat	I: 70-75% THR D: 40-50 min jogging continuously F: 5-7/week C: Flat or hills
Monday	30 min	30 min hill course	40 min	40 min hill course
Tuesday	35 min	35 min flat course	45 min	45 min flat course
Wednesday	40 min	40 min flat course	50 min	50 min flat course
Thursday	35 min	35 min hill course	45 min	45 min hill course
Friday	Rest, strength, or other mode	Rest, strength, or other mode	Rest, strength, or other mode	Rest, strength, or other mode
Saturday	40 min	40 min hill course	50 min	50 min hill course
Sunday	35 min	35 min flat course	40 min	40 min flat course
	Improvement phase			
	Weeks 5-9	**Weeks 10-14**	**Weeks 15-19**	**Weeks 20-24**
Exercise components	I: 75-80% THR D: 40-50 min jogging continuously F: 5-7/week C: Flat	I: 75-80% THR D: 40-50 min jogging continuously F: 5-7/week C: Flat or hills	I: 75-80% THR D: 50-60 min jogging continuously F: 5-7/week C: Flat	I: 75-80% THR D: 50-60 min jogging continuously F: 5-7/week C: Flat or hills
Monday	40 min	40 min hill course	50 min	50 min hill course
Tuesday	45 min	45 min flat course	55 min	55 min flat course
Wednesday	50 min	50 min flat course	60 min	60 min flat course
Thursday	45 min	45 min hill course	55 min	55 min hill course
Friday	Rest, strength, or other mode	Rest, strength, or other mode	Rest, strength, or other mode	Rest, strength, or other mode
Saturday	50 min	50 min hill course	60 min	60 min hill course
Sunday	40 min	40 min flat course	50 min	50 min flat course
	Maintenance phase			
	Weeks 25+			
Exercise components	I: 70-85% THR D: 40-60 min jogging continuously F: 3/week C: Flat or hills			
Monday-Sunday	Combine the above components to achieve 70-85% THR to maintain training effect.			

I = intensity; D = duration; F = frequency; C = course; THR = target heart rate
Always exercise on alternate days if possible, and always incorporate a rest day.

Cycling

Cycling is another excellent mode of exercise. Cycling recruits large muscles from the lower extremities as well as the core muscles of your trunk. Cycling is a very low-impact aerobic exercise ideally suited for individuals with arthritic joints. Indoor cycling is a good choice of aerobic exercise if you have EIA, asthma, allergic rhinitis, or other physical allergies. As with running and walking, cycling will improve lung function and your exercise tolerance. Initial and advanced cycling programs are outlined in tables 3.11 and 3.12 on pages 71 and 72.

Equipment, Medication, and Environment

Indoor and outdoor cycling each have distinct advantages and disadvantages. Cycling indoors allows you to exercise in a climate-controlled environment with ideal temperature and humidity. Also, many allergens exist outdoors that simply do not exist indoors. If you are allergic to ragweed, tree pollen, flower pollen, or other grasses, exercising indoors may minimize your contact with these allergens. However, if you have difficulty with dust mites, animal dander, or molds, indoor cycling may not provide less exposure to allergens. A television or radio can provide entertainment to combat boredom with stationary indoor cycling.

Stationary bikes come in two basic types, erect or recumbent. Either type of stationary bike will work well. The seat should be positioned so that your leg is slightly flexed when the pedal is at its farthest point from your body. Clothing should be light, loose, and synthetic to facilitate movement and heat exchange. A helmet is not necessary if you are riding a stationary bike. Always take your medications before exercise and have your rescue inhaler handy. Athletic shoes should be worn for stationary cycling, but use your running or walking shoes only for those activities. Stationary bikes provide easy control of intensity. Most bikes have a method of checking your heart rate and easily adjustable RPM or resistance levels. Try using a stationary bike for at least a month before considering hitting the road.

Speaking of hitting the road, outdoor cycling is one of the more enjoyable aerobic activities. Some cyclists like the scenery, some like the sense of freedom, and some are just bike technology "junkies," but they all love to hit the road. The last thing you probably want to do on your bike is actually hit the road. If you are not accustomed to cycling, start with short trips during less busy travel times and use less traveled roads. Wind and wind currents created by cycling will dry and reduce the temperature of your lungs while you breathe. For this reason, outdoor cycling can propose an increased risk for EIA or asthma. You may minimize risk by cycling on warmer, more humid days or wearing a mask. Cycling during low-pollen-count days while wearing a mask may reduce your allergen exposure. You are part of the road and all the dangers that go with being part of the road, so ride defensively.

Buying a bike can be exciting and confusing. Try buying or borrowing a beginner road or hybrid bike. Visit your local bicycle shop to ensure proper fit. If you are borrowing a bike, make sure you take it to the shop for a tune-up. When you buy your bike, you must buy a helmet, no exceptions. The helmet and the bike are the only essential pieces of equipment. I participate in triathlons and road races, and my helmet never leaves my head until I'm done riding and my bike is in the rack. You are outdoors, so dress with appropriate layers and sunscreen to prevent solar urticaria, cold urticaria, heat illness, exposure, and sun damage to your skin. I recommend riding in an empty parking lot to get familiar with braking and changing gears. You will use your gears to adjust intensity of your ride. Carry your rescue inhaler, other medications, and a mobile phone in your saddle bag.

Cycling Programs

When beginning the cycling programs shown in tables 3.11 and 3.12, you should be able to walk comfortably for 20 to 30 minutes at 40 to 50 percent of your target heart rate. Start at low resistance, and gradually increase the duration and intensity over a month. The program gradually increases the intensity and duration with varying resistance. As with walking and running, it is best to incorporate strength training or another mode of exercise in the program. Once you reach the maintenance phase, you will have more freedom to design your own program within the guidelines. This is the phase where you should consider cycling outdoors. Shifting gears or choosing a hilly course will vary your resistance. If you experience asthma symptoms or EIA twice a week, see your physician and drop back to the previous level of cycling or change your exercise environment. If your fitness level is very high, you may consider starting around the weeks 20 to 24 exercise level.

Swimming

The previous modes of aerobic exercise are all excellent activities to improve your quality of life and fitness. Swimming certainly fits in the same category as those exercises but is superior when compared to those exercises in terms of asthmogenicity. Several studies over the past 20 years have shown that the body undergoes similar adaptations when stimulated by swimming, cycling, running, or walking (Clark 1993). These same studies compared the number of asthma or EIA exacerbations among individuals starting various exercise programs, and swimming produced the least number. Also, when compared to other indoor modes of aerobic exercise, swimming resulted in fewer complications from asthma and EIA. Most of these studies were performed in a heated indoor pool. Increased lung capacity, increased aerobic capacity, reduced exercise-induced bronchoconstriction, lower blood pressure, lower pulse rate, and improved

Table 3.11 Initial Cycling Program

	Initial phase			
	Week 1	**Week 2**	**Week 3**	**Week 4**
Exercise components	I: 50% THR D: 20 min F: 3/week R: Low	I: 50% THR D: 20-25 min F: 3/week R: Low	I: 55% THR D: 25-30 min F: 3-5/week R: Low	I: 55% THR D: 30-35 min F: 3-5/week R: Low
Monday	20 min	20 min	25 min	30 min
Tuesday	Rest	Rest	25 min	30 min
Wednesday	Strength or other mode	Strength or other mode	Rest, strength, or other mode	Rest, strength, or other mode
Thursday	20 min	20 min	30 min	35 min
Friday	Rest	Rest	Rest	Rest
Saturday	20 min	25 min	30 min	35 min
Sunday	Rest, strength, or other mode	Rest, strength, or other mode	Rest, strength, or other mode	Rest, strength, or other mode
	Improvement phase			
	Weeks 5-9	**Weeks 10-14**	**Weeks 15-19**	**Weeks 20-24**
Exercise components	I: 60-65% THR D: 30-40 min F: 5/week R: Low	I: 60-65% THR D: 35-45 min F: 5/week R: Low/med	I: 65-70% THR D: 40-50 min F: 5/week R: Low	I: 65-70% THR D: 40-50 min F: 5/week R: Low/med
Monday	30 min	35 min med	40 min	40 min med
Tuesday	35 min	40 min low	45 min	45 min low
Wednesday	Rest, strength, or other mode	Rest, strength, or other mode	Rest, strength, or other mode	Rest, strength, or other mode
Thursday	40 min	45 min low	50 min	50 min low
Friday	Rest, strength, or other mode	Rest, strength, or other mode	Rest, strength, or other mode	Rest, strength, or other mode
Saturday	40 min	45 min med	50 min	50 min med
Sunday	35 min	40 min med	45 min	45 min med
	Maintenance phase			
	Weeks 25+			
Exercise components	I: 70-80% THR D: 40-60 min F: 3/week R: Low, medium, or high C: Indoor or outdoor			
Monday-Sunday	Combine the above components to achieve 70-80% THR to maintain training effect.			

I = intensity; D = duration; F = frequency; C = course; THR = target heart rate; R = resistance
Always exercise on alternate days if possible, and always incorporate a rest day.

Table 3.12 Advanced Cycling Program

	Initial phase			
	Week 1	**Week 2**	**Week 3**	**Week 4**
Exercise components	I: 70-80% THR D: 40-60 min F: 5/week R: Med	I: 70-80% THR D: 50-60 min F: 5/week R: Med	I: 70-80% THR D: 50-60 min F: 5/week R: Med/high	I: 70-80% THR D: 60 min F: 5/week R: Med/high
Monday	40 min	50 min	50 min med	60 min med
Tuesday	40 min	50 min	50 min high	60 min high
Wednesday	60 min	60 min	60 min med	60 min med
Thursday	Rest, strength, or other mode	Rest, strength, or other mode	Rest, strength, or other mode	Rest, strength, or other mode
Friday	40 min	50 min	50 min med	60 min med
Saturday	60 min	60 min	60 min high	60 min high
Sunday	Rest, strength, or other mode	Rest, strength, or other mode	Rest, strength, or other mode	Rest, strength, or other mode
	Improvement phase			
	Weeks 5-9	**Weeks 10-14**	**Weeks 15-19**	**Weeks 20-24**
Exercise components	I: 80-85% THR D: 60-80 min F: 5/week R: med, interval, and hill climb	I: 80-85% THR D: 60-80 min F: 5/week R: med, interval, and hill climb	I: 80-85% THR D: 60-90 min F: 5/week R: high, interval, and hill climb	I: 80-85% THR D: 60-90 min F: 5/week R: high, interval, and hill climb
Monday	60 min hill climb	60 min interval	80 min hill climb	90 min interval
Tuesday	80 min interval	80 min hill climb	80 min interval	90 min hill climb
Wednesday	60 min med	60 min med	60 min high	60 min high
Thursday	Rest, strength, or other mode	Rest, strength, or other mode	Rest, strength, or other mode	Rest, strength, or other mode
Friday	60 min med	60 min med	60 min high	60 min high
Saturday	80 min interval	80 min hill climb	90 min hill climb	90 min interval
Sunday	Rest, strength, or other mode	Rest, strength, or other mode	Rest, strength, or other mode	Rest, strength, or other mode
	Maintenance phase			
	Weeks 25+			
Exercise components	I: 80-85% THR D: 90 min F: 3/week R: high, interval, and hill climb			
Monday-Sunday	Combine the above components to achieve 80-85% THR in order to maintain training effect.			

I = intensity; D = duration; F = frequency; C = course; THR = target heart rate; R = resistance
Always exercise on alternate days if possible, and always incorporate a rest day.

exercise tolerance were all documented among participants enrolled in various swimming programs. I have spent a lot of personal time swimming in public pools, health clubs, and other gymnasiums filled with people enjoying the benefits of swimming. From children to elderly people, men and women, and chronically ill to healthy, almost anyone can start and benefit from a swim program.

Equipment, Medication, and Environment

The warm, humid environment of an indoor swimming pool is an ideal setting for exercise with asthma, EIA, or allergic rhinitis. I was recently covering a high school football game and was called to the natatorium to treat a high school swimmer for an asthma attack. An asthma attack can still occur in an ideal environment, so you should always have your rescue inhaler handy. If you have a rare condition such as chlorine sensitivity or aquagenic urticaria, a swimming program is not a good idea. Remember to hydrate; even though you are surrounded by water, you are still losing sweat. I recommend taking a swimming lesson at your local park district, health club, or YMCA before starting the program. Lessons will improve your stroke efficiency, and you will enjoy swimming much more. You must take lessons if you are a very inexperienced swimmer. Open water swimming should be reserved for those who are very fit and very experienced swimmers. Always swim in a lifeguard-supervised area or with a partner who knows CPR. A swimming program is not ideally suited for those with exercise-induced anaphylaxis because of the risk of drowning.

Swimming Programs

A swimming program can be quite flexible and variable. Incorporating different strokes, kickboards, and intervals can provide enough variety to keep the program interesting. Sedentary individuals should start in the initial phase of the swim program (see table 3.13). Moderately fit individuals may start at the improvement phase of the initial swimming program, and very fit individuals can use the advanced program in table 3.14. Your asthma and EIA should be under good control before starting the program. The same guidelines should be applied to progressing from one phase to the next. Determining the intensity of your swim session may be difficult because your pulse may be lower than normal in the water and it is difficult to measure your pulse while swimming. I recommend using the RPE scale to measure your intensity (see page 50). Swim sessions start with short intervals and progress to longer, continuous sessions. Eventually long, continuous sessions are combined with intervals. I leave it up to you to change the stroke, but you should use a kickboard to condition your lower legs at least once a week. You should also incorporate a dry-land, weight training session for strength and endurance.

Table 3.13 Initial Swimming Program

	Initial phase			
	Week 1	**Week 2**	**Week 3**	**Week 4**
Exercise components	I: Light D: 20 min F: 3/week	I: Light D: 20-30 min F: 3/week	I: Moderate D: 20-30 min F: 3/week	I: Moderate D: 30 min F: 3/week
Monday	4 5-min intervals	2 10-min intervals	1 20- and 10-min interval	30 min continuous
Tuesday	Rest	Rest	Rest	Rest
Wednesday	4 5-min intervals	1 10- and 15-min interval	1 20- and 10-min interval	30 min continuous
Thursday	Rest	Rest	Rest	Rest
Friday	2 10-min intervals	2 15-min intervals	30 min continuous	30 min continuous
Saturday	Strength	Strength	Strength	Strength
Sunday	Rest	Rest	Rest	Rest
	Improvement phase			
	Weeks 5-9	**Weeks 10-14**	**Weeks 15-19**	**Weeks 20-24**
Exercise components	I: Moderate to hard D: 30-40 min F: 3-5/week	I: Moderate to hard D: 40 min F: 3-5/week	I: Hard to very hard D: 40-50 min F: 3-5/week	I: Hard to very hard D: 50 min F: 3-5/week
Monday	35 min continuous	40 min continuous	40 min continuous hard	50 min continuous hard
Tuesday	Rest	Rest	Rest	Rest
Wednesday	40 min continuous	40 min continuous	40 min continuous hard	50 min continuous hard
Thursday	3 10-min intervals hard	4 10-min intervals hard	5 10-min intervals very hard	5 10-min intervals very hard
Friday	Rest or strength	Rest or strength	Rest or strength	Rest or strength
Saturday	Kickboard 3 10-min intervals	Kickboard 3 10-min intervals	Kickboard 3 10-min intervals	Kickboard 3 10-min intervals
Sunday	40 min continuous	40 min continuous	50 min continuous hard	50 min continuous hard
	Maintenance phase			
	Weeks 25+			
Exercise components	I: Hard to very hard D: 40-60 min F: 3/week Continuous or interval			
Monday-Sunday	Combine the above components to achieve hard to very hard intensity to maintain training effect.			

I = intensity; D = duration; F = frequency
Always exercise on alternate days if possible, and always incorporate a rest day.

Table 3.14 Advanced Swimming Program

Initial phase				
	Week 1	**Week 2**	**Week 3**	**Week 4**
Exercise components	I: Hard to very hard D: 40-60 min F: 5/week Continuous, interval, and kickboard	I: Hard to very hard D: 40-60 min F: 5/week Continuous, interval, and kickboard	I: Hard to very hard D: 40-60 min F: 5/week Continuous, interval, and kickboard	I: Hard to very hard D: 40-60 min F: 5/week Continuous, interval, and kickboard
Monday	50 min hard continuous	50 min hard continuous	60 min hard continuous	60 min hard continuous
Tuesday	Rest, strength, or other mode	Rest, strength, or other mode	Rest, strength, or other mode	Rest, strength, or other mode
Wednesday	40 min very hard continuous	40 min very hard continuous	45 min very hard continuous	45 min very hard continuous
Thursday	4 10-min intervals hard	4 10-min intervals hard-very hard-hard-very hard	3 15-min intervals hard-very hard-hard	3 15-min intervals very hard-hard-very hard
Friday	Rest, strength, or other mode	Rest, strength, or other mode	Rest, strength, or other mode	Rest, strength, or other mode
Saturday	3 15-min intervals hard kickboard	3 15-min intervals hard-very hard-hard kickboard	5 10-min intervals hard kickboard	5 10-min intervals alternate hard-very hard kickboard
Sunday	60 min hard continuous	60 min hard continuous	60 min very hard continuous	60 min very hard continuous
Improvement phase				
	Weeks 5-9	**Weeks 10-14**	**Weeks 15-19**	**Weeks 20-24**
Exercise components	I: Hard to very hard D: 45-60 min F: 5/week Continuous, interval, upper body only, and kickboard	I: Hard to very hard D: 45-60 min F: 5/week Continuous, interval, upper body only, and kickboard	I: Hard to very hard D: 45-80 min F: 5/week Continuous, interval, upper body only, and kickboard	I: Hard to very hard D: 45-80 min F: 5/week Continuous, interval, upper body only, and kickboard
Monday	60 min very hard continuous	60 min very hard continuous	60 min very hard continuous	60 min very hard continuous

(continued)

Table 3.14 *(continued)*

	Improvement phase			
	Weeks 5-9	**Weeks 10-14**	**Weeks 15-19**	**Weeks 20-24**
Tuesday	Rest, strength, or other mode	Rest, strength, or other mode	Rest, strength, or other mode	Rest, strength, or other mode
Wednesday	50 min very hard continuous	50 min very hard continuous	50 min very hard continuous	50 min very hard continuous
Thursday	3 15-min intervals hard alternate upper body-kickboard	3 15-min intervals hard-very hard-hard upper body only	3 15-min intervals very hard alternate upper body-kickboard	3 15-min intervals hard-very hard-hard upper body only
Friday	Rest, strength, or other mode	Rest, strength, or other mode	Rest, strength, or other mode	Rest, strength, or other mode
Saturday	5 10-min intervals hard alternate upper body-kickboard	5 10-min intervals alternate hard-very hard alternate upper body-kickboard	4 15-min intervals hard alternate upper body-kickboard	4 15-min intervals very hard alternate upper body-kickboard
Sunday	60 min very hard continuous	60 min very hard continuous	80 min hard continuous	80 min very hard continuous
	Maintenance phase			
	Weeks 25+			
Exercise components	I: Hard to very hard D: 45-80 min F: 3/week Continuous, interval, upper body only, and kickboard			
Monday-Sunday	Combine the above components to achieve hard to very hard intensity to maintain training effect.			

I = intensity; D = duration; F = frequency
Always exercise on alternate days if possible, and always incorporate a rest day.

Summary

Aerobic exercise will improve your fitness. To that end, I am sure you understand the importance of an aerobic exercise program in treating and improving asthma and EIA. These exercise programs are guidelines to improving your fitness and are not meant to replace the guidance of your personal physician, physical therapist, or athletic trainer. Always remember to use your medications as directed and have them available if you need them. Careful preparation for exercise will ensure a safe and enjoyable exercise program. I always advocate incorporating different modes of aerobic exercise in an exercise program to combat boredom. Feel free to add or remove different modes of exercise or change your exercise routine to keep it enjoyable. Before you make changes, make sure your asthma, EIA, and allergies are under good control. Don't forget about flexibility and strength training; they are just as important as aerobic exercise. Have a great exercise experience, and stay fit.

ACTION PLAN:

TARGETING ASTHMA THROUGH AEROBIC EXERCISE

☐ Explore the many types of aerobic activity to find the ones you enjoy most.

☐ Use your $\dot{V}O_2$max and heart rate to calculate the appropriate exercise intensity for your program.

☐ Aim to get 20 to 60 minutes of continuous or intermittent aerobic activity throughout the day, 3 to 5 days a week.

☐ Plan sufficient warm-up and cool-down sessions, including using your inhaler before the warm-up.

☐ Use the sample walking, running, cycling, and swimming programs given in this chapter, or tailor them to fit your needs.

☐ Make sure to keep your inhaler with you during exercise!

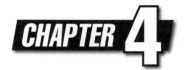

CHAPTER 4

BUILDING STRENGTH AND FLEXIBILITY

Jeffrey M. Mjaanes

W hen we think of exercise, we think of fitness. But what does it mean to be fit? The term *fitness* takes on different meanings to different people. However, many experts have described three basic elements that are common to the idea of fitness: cardiovascular conditioning, flexibility, and strength, the so-called fitness triangle. Chapter 3 focused on aerobic, or cardiovascular exercise; this chapter discusses strength and flexibility.

First, we must clarify some terms. Many people confuse strength training with weightlifting or bodybuilding. Beginners may imagine muscle-bound men and women pumping iron in the gym, become disillusioned with the idea of lifting weights, and decide that strength training is not right for them. Therefore, some definitions are in order.

The term *strength training* is synonymous with *resistance training;* it means using progressive, repetitive resistance methods to increase one's ability to exert or resist force. Strength training includes the use of free weights, weight machines, rubber tubing, body weight, medicine balls, or other resistance devices. Weightlifting is technically a competitive Olympic sport testing maximum lifting ability through such techniques as the clean and snatch. In common vernacular, weightlifting may also refer to the use of free weights or machines at a gym; however, this definition still does not reflect the entire variety of modalities available with strength training. Powerlifting is also a competitive sport testing limited maximum lifting ability, such as the deadlift. Bodybuilding is a competition of muscle size, symmetry, and definition. Neither powerlifting nor bodybuilding focus on low-resistance strength training or aerobic exercise to improve overall fitness.

In general, *fitness* refers to a general state of health in which muscle and tendon integrity, bone mass, glucose tolerance, fat-free mass, and resting metabolic rate are at optimal levels. Furthermore, all of these fitness components can be improved or maintained by muscular fitness. The term *muscular fitness* is used to describe integration of muscular strength and muscular endurance. Muscular strength refers to the maximal force that can be generated by a muscle or muscle group at a given velocity, such as a maximum bench press or lifting a heavy box at home. Muscular endurance is the ability of a muscle group to perform repeated contractions over a time period sufficient to cause muscular fatigue, such as the maximum number of push-ups that can be done without rest. Another way to define muscular endurance is the ability of a muscle or muscle group to maintain a specific percentage of maximum voluntary contraction for a prolonged time, such as when you carry groceries in from the car. In most resistance training programs, we work to achieve and balance both muscular strength and endurance.

Despite the emphasis on improving strength and endurance, we cannot overlook the importance of flexibility. Flexibility is the ability to relax and stretch a muscle. Maintaining muscle flexibility is the third component of the fitness triangle and should be incorporated into every training program.

Strength Training

In addition to purely improving strength, participation in a regular strength training program has numerous positive benefits on the human body. Working your muscles through resistance training increases circulation to muscle cells, increasing muscle fiber size and improving the integrity of your muscle-tendon units. Stronger muscles, in turn, absorb stresses otherwise passed on to joints, thus reducing injury- and arthritis-associated pain.

Weight training also builds lean muscle mass and thus increases your resting metabolic rate. With a higher metabolic rate, you will burn calories much more efficiently and, in the end, further improve your overall body composition, with lower body fat and higher lean muscle mass. Resistance training has also been shown to improve bone mass and bone mineral density, which is critical to the prevention of osteoporosis and fragility fractures. Blood lipid profiles also improve, potentially decreasing the risk for heart attacks and strokes.

Combining strength training with some sort of aerobic exercise can remarkably improve cardiorespiratory fitness, further lowering risk for heart disease. For those individuals with allergic disease, in particular asthma, the improvement in cardiovascular fitness may lead to better overall health and asthma control. Many people with asthma are afraid to exercise strenuously because they fear they will worsen their asthma. However, if one's asthma is under adequate control, exercise can generally be done safely. In fact, the positive overall health benefits of regular exercise far outweigh the potential risk of an asthma attack in those with well-controlled asthma. In addition, it is well established that a risk is associated between obesity and cardiovascular disease and asthma. In my practice, I usually encourage overweight and obese teens to begin increasing activities by strength training. These adolescents tend to be strong and can make definite gains in strength and self-esteem, motivating them

Benefits of Strength Training

▸ Improved muscle circulation

▸ Improved musculotendinous integrity

▸ Increased lean muscle mass

▸ Improved overall body composition

▸ Higher resting metabolic rate

▸ Improved bone mass and bone mineral density

▸ Improved blood lipid profile

▸ Improved cardiorespiratory fitness

▸ Improved self-esteem

toward more aerobic exercise in the future. In fact, perhaps the greatest effect of strength training is the psychological impact and improved self-esteem, which motivate us to continue striving to meet our goals.

Some people ask, "How can lifting a few weights do all this for my body?" It works this way: Strength training overloads the muscle and microscopically causes muscle breakdown. During the rest period that follows, the body repairs the damage by sending blood and nutrients to the exhausted muscle cells. At the same time, each exercise you perform also teaches the muscle how to respond to force, and it recruits more muscle fibers to resist that force. Strength training increases muscle fiber size; muscle contractile strength; as well as bone, tendon, and ligament tensile strength. This process results in stronger, larger muscles, although the extent of which depends on your age, your gender, and your strength training goals. Children and adolescents who have not completed puberty have insufficient levels of the male sex hormone testosterone in their blood and have difficulty gaining large muscle size. Mature males, both adolescents and adults, make size gains because of the amount of testosterone in their blood. Women have less testosterone than men. This relative lack of testosterone explains why children and women make strength gains primarily through neuromuscular training and muscle fiber recruitment, while men make gains through muscle hypertrophy (increased actual muscle size). In other words, children and women retrain their muscle fibers to actually exert more force through improved muscle coordination and internal changes within the muscle. In any case both women and men, young and old, can benefit from regular strength training.

Strength Training for a Lifetime

Many people think they are too old to lift weights, and many parents think their children are too young to strength train. The truth is, when one is old enough to understand the techniques and follow simple exercise plans, one is ready to weight train—and one is never too old to train.

Children

Multiple studies show that children as young as 8 years old can not only safely engage in a strength training program but also reap the benefits such as increased strength and improved self-esteem (Faigenbaum 2000). The overall key to safe strength training for children and adolescents is supervision. Children must learn proper technique for each exercise, maintain strict form throughout the exercise, have direct supervision by an adult educated in youth resistance training, and focus on light to moderate weights. If young athletes follow these guidelines, studies show their risk of injury is minimal. In fact, the only serious and fatal injuries from weightlifting in this age group have been adolescent boys lifting weights, mainly the bench press, at home unsupervised. Besides this scenario, strength training is actually safer than most contact sports.

Children actually do get stronger, not through testosterone-induced increases in muscle size, but through neuromuscular changes in muscle unit recruitment. Do these increases in strength translate into improved sport performance? If the sport the child plays is one that depends on strength, such as football or wrestling, then strength training may have a positive effect on performance. However, strength training will not alter talent or skill and therefore is unlikely to have a major impact on sport performance.

The time-old myth that lifting weights will stunt your growth appears to be a great overstatement at best. Studies fail to show that kids who engage in regular strength training end up with shorter adult heights than peers. Lifting light to moderate weights does not seem to have a negative effect on a developing child's bones or growth plates (sites in long bones from which extremity growth occurs). Nevertheless, children who are still growing and have not reached the end of puberty, or skeletal maturity, need to be especially careful to use lighter weights with strict form and avoid lifting very heavy weights, especially with poor form.

Older Adults

Human peak muscular strength occurs between 25 and 30 years of age. After age 30, both men and women start to lose lean muscle mass. Decreased physical activity will likely hasten the process. The older you are, the more you need to start resistance training. Older men and women may lead lives that are more sedentary, and the lack of regular exercise leads to generalized muscle atrophy and weakness. Unfortunately a vicious cycle of increased risk for injury results, causing even less activity and increased muscle weakness. Improved strength helps older individuals maintain their mobility and their ability to perform activities of daily living.

Another benefit of strength training is improved bone health. The improvement in bone mineral density occurs in all ages, from adolescents to middle-aged to older individuals. Bone mass decreases by about .5 percent a year after the age of 40, and this decline in bone mineral density predisposes the elderly to increased risk of fragility fractures of the hip and spine (Kohrt et al. 2004). These fractures, in particular those in the hip, can be catastrophic. The mortality rate for elderly individuals in the first year following a hip fracture approaches 20 percent (Kohrt et al. 2004). To maintain strong bones throughout adulthood, you must ensure a diet rich in calcium and engage in a regular strength training program. Even seniors can safely strength train and, in fact, they will benefit greatly from the increased strength and increased mobility. Before starting a strength training plan, especially if you are an older adult, you should see a physician for a complete physical to ensure that you can begin safely.

Types of Resistance Training

In general, muscle contractions can be divided into two main groups: dynamic and static. Eccentric contractions, in which the muscle lengthens as force is applied, represent a type of dynamic exercise. The other primary type of dynamic exercise is a concentric contraction such as a typical biceps curl where the muscle contracts and shortens as force is applied. Dynamic exercises are usually isotonic in nature, meaning that the muscle contracts with movement against a natural resistance. Isokinetic exercises are ones in which the muscle contracts against a force at a constant speed. Diagnostic strength equipment implements isokinetic tension to measure strength at varying joint angles. All types of resistance training are fine for developing strength, but most physiotherapists recommend dynamic exercises because they most closely imitate natural muscle movements. In fact, ACSM's newest exercise guidelines recommend performing 3 seconds of a concentric phase and 3 seconds of an eccentric phase into each strengthening exercise repetition (ACSM 2005).

Static exercises are isometric, meaning the length of the muscle stays constant while the muscle is undergoing contraction. For example, tighten your abdominal muscles and hold your breath for a few seconds. The muscle is not changing length as it would during a sit-up or a crunch, but it still contracts. In general, isometric or static tension exercises are not as preferable as dynamic exercises because isometric training does not place the muscle or adjacent joint through a full range of motion.

Two basic types of movement exist to dynamically elicit a muscle contraction: open chain and closed chain. An open-chain exercise is one in which the end segment of the exercised limb, the end not supporting the weight, is not fixed. Most isolated exercises are open-chain movements. An example of an open-chain exercise is a leg extension machine at the gym for quadriceps strengthening, where the foot is free and not fixed. A closed-chain exercise is one in which the end segment of the exercised limb, the end supporting the weight, is fixed. Most compound exercises are closed-chain movements. An example of a closed-chain exercise is a wall slide for quadriceps strengthening, where the person stands with the back against the wall and slowly bends at the knee and waist until reaching a squatting position and then returns to standing. In this case the feet are fixed against the floor. In general, closed-chain exercises are more functional and therefore are preferable to open-chain exercises.

Putting Together a Plan

Whether you have been training for a while or are just looking to begin, a quick refresher on the basic components of a strength training program can be helpful. Beginners may need an introduction to the basic layout of a training routine, the equipment, and proper form. More advanced weight trainers can use the following information to spice up their workout and maybe try some new exercises while reviewing their technique.

Goals

When you are ready to put together a strength training plan, you need to decide whether your goal is to improve strength, endurance, or both. People who are interested in adding lean muscle mass and getting stronger will formulate a different workout plan than those who want to increase their stamina and endurance. Some people may have other objectives as well. Many people start an exercise program because they are interested in gaining or losing weight, while others simply want to maintain their current weight but still work on strength or endurance. Injured athletes, recreational or otherwise, want to regain strength and range of motion during rehabilitation from injury. Frequently those with injuries will be in a tightly organized strength training program that emphasizes neuromuscular control with many repetitions of very low resistance several times a day. Table 4.1 shows general ranges for the components of the program for different goals.

Intensity

The intensity of a strength workout generally refers to the amount of weight or resistance used. Your workout intensity will depend on your goals and your starting point. For maintenance of muscle tone and endurance, one usually lifts light-moderate weights, performing multiple sets of many (10-15) repetitions without major increases in the amount of weight or resistance. For those interested in increasing muscle mass, the focus will be on increasing resistance through a heavier weight range with fewer repetitions. Obviously beginners will start with light weights and advance gradually to moderate weights.

Table 4.1   Resistance Training Continuum

Goals	Endurance/strength	Strength
Intensity	40-60% of 1RM	> 85% of 1RM
Reps	12-20	8-10
Sets	3-5	3-4
Frequency	2-3 times/week	3-4 times/week

Adapted, by permission, from A.L. Millar, 2003, *Action plan for arthritis* (Champaign, IL: Human Kinetics), 81.

Many methods exist for determining intensity for a strength training program. The "gold standard" of dynamic strength testing is the 1 repetition maximum (1RM), which is the heaviest weight you can lift only once, but not twice, using good form. The primary disadvantage of the 1RM is that you really need spotters or a training buddy to help you control the weight to prevent potentially serious injury. You should not attempt to lift a 1RM alone.

You can also estimate your 1RM by using a fairly simple formula. First, find a weight that you can lift at least 10 times but not more. Then, take this weight and divide by .75 to get an estimate of your 1RM. This formula assumes you will be able to lift at least 75 percent of your maximum. For example, if you can bench press 100 pounds 10 times, divide 100 by .75 and round up to get a 1RM of 135 pounds. Then you can use the 1RM to make adjustments to the intensity of your individual workouts based on your starting point and objectives (see Sample Strength Programs on page 105).

Another means of finding how much you can lift is to begin with a very low weight that is quite easy and gradually increase the weight until you can barely lift a certain amount 10 times while still maintaining strict form. This method is probably the most common form for determining intensity because it is simple and can be done without assistance. Nevertheless, you should still use a spotter as you progress into the heavier weight ranges, especially if you are inexperienced in the weight room.

Progression

To gain strength, you need to progressively add resistance. Basically, you can increase resistance by either adding weight each set or increasing the number of repetitions each set. The easiest means of determining how to advance your workout is based on form. Because strict form with controlled movements is also the key to avoiding injury, it makes sense that this is the best way to make strength gains as well. So, increase the number of reps in a set or add weight when you are able to complete a predetermined number of repetitions while still maintaining strict form easily without strain. For example, once you can perform 10 to 12 biceps curls with a 10-pound dumbbell while using proper form and technique, then increase to a 12-pound dumbbell for the next set and continue at this weight until you can complete 10 to 12 repetitions again. Another method would be to increase the number of repetitions from, say, 10 to 15 when you can maintain strict form, and then increase the weight by 5 or 10 pounds at the next session and start at 8 repetitions. Whichever method you choose, when you increase the weight or the number of repetitions, you should do so by no more than 10 percent each week to avoid muscle fatigue. Increasing resistance and intensity too quickly is a common reason for injuries, some potentially serious.

The example just used applies mostly to free weights. If you are working on a strength training routine at home, you can still advance your workout in a number of ways. If you are working with rubber tubing, you can increase the resistance of the rubber bands to the next color (most are color-coded for different levels of resistance). If you are mainly using your own body weight for resistance, you can use creative ways to augment your workout. With push-ups, for example, you can increase the number of repetitions or make the exercise more challenging by placing your feet on a step and doing the push-up at an incline. Again, remember to increase your intensity gradually to avoid muscle fatigue and injury. A key to remember at the gym or at home is to keep shaking up your routine. Variations will keep your workout fresh and prevent you from hitting a plateau.

Frequency

I am frequently asked, "How often should I work out?" The frequency of your workout depends on several factors, including your schedule, location and accessibility of the workout facility and, most importantly, your goals for strength training. If your goal is to build strength, then focus on a low to moderate number of repetitions (8-10) of high-resistance exercises, approximately 80 percent of your 1RM. Bodybuilders and competitive weightlifters train 5 to 6 days a week, but most of us should aim to train 3 days a week with a day of rest in between. If you want to simply tone up for muscular endurance, you will also want to use more repetitions (15-20) and less resistance. For the general population, ACSM recommends 2 to 3 days a week of resistance training. ACSM also recommends 8 to 10 exercises to work major muscle groups, with 3 to 20 repetitions per set (ACSM 2005).

You will likely want to train different body parts on the same day because when you perform an exercise for one muscle, you often employ other muscle groups to complete the movement. For example, some people choose to train the biceps and back on the same day, legs and shoulders on the same day, and chest and triceps on the same day. When you perform a bench press, you activate your pectoral muscles as well as your triceps and some anterior deltoid fibers. Another example is the latissimus pull-down, in which you use your latissimus dorsi muscle as well as the biceps. Therefore, training triceps and chest or biceps and back the same day allows you to still leave a day in between for rest.

Other strength trainers tend to train opposing muscle groups the same day. Opposing muscle groups are also called agonist-antagonist muscles. For example, the biceps and the triceps are agonist-antagonist muscles because one acts to flex and the other to extend the elbow joint. Another example of such opposing muscles is the hamstring and the quadriceps in the thigh; the hamstring flexes the knee while the quadriceps extends the knee. In my experience, training opposing groups the same day tends to fatigue that body part more rapidly and leaves me feeling weaker after my workout, but others enjoy dedicating one day to arms and another day to legs. Choose what best works for you.

Most people perform multiple exercises for each body part. Performing two or three different exercises for each muscle group is a good idea. Because you will be training two or three different body parts the same day, you will end up performing roughly 6 to 10 exercises each session. Aim to perform 2 to 4 sets for each exercise of 8 to 12 repetitions each. Make sure to leave time in between each set to rest the muscle for the next set and still maintain proper form. Leaving less than 1 minute between sets leads to earlier fatigue, while lifters who rest more than 3 minutes between sets tend to become bored with their workout quickly. A rest period of 1 or 2 minutes between sets is ideal—and the perfect time for a water break! Be efficient in your workout, and do not feel you have to stay in the gym 2 hours to reap the benefits of a strengthening program. According to ACSM, any exercise program lasting more than 1 hour tends to lead to fatigue and higher dropout rates (ACSM 2005).

Tips for Strength Training

- ▸ Aim to work out 2 or 3 days a week with a day of rest in between.
- ▸ Perform multiple exercises (2-4) for different muscle groups (total 8-10).
- ▸ Do 3 sets for each exercise.
- ▸ Aim to perform 8 to 12 repetitions for each set.
- ▸ Rest 1 to 3 minutes between sets.
- ▸ Train one or two body parts each session (e.g., chest and triceps).
- ▸ Set aside an hour for your workout.
- ▸ Add resistance when you can do 10 to 12 repetitions easily with proper form.
- ▸ Include cardiovascular exercise and stretching in your routine.
- ▸ Warm up before your workout and cool down afterward.

Choosing a Location for Strength Training

So, you have already committed yourself to strength training and have an idea of your goals and how to plan your routine. At this stage, another question you need to ask yourself is, Should you work out at home or at a fitness facility. The location question is important since both settings usually involve significant expense. Nevertheless, low-cost options do exist for both locales. The answer to the question depends on what is right for you as an individual, your likes and dislikes, your budget and transportation.

Your house can serve as an ideal location for working out. The advantages are that you do not have to rely on transportation, you may keep the initial costs low, and you can work out in the privacy of your own home. You may choose to invest in weight training equipment and free weights and set up a complete home gym. However, inexpensive options exist, especially if you are just starting to work with resistance training. For relatively low initial cost you can purchase handheld or cuff weights and rubber tubing, or you can use your own body weight (which is free!) and do push-ups, pull-ups, and wall slides. With your body weight, rubber tubing, inexpensive small weights, and a medicine ball, you can arrange an ideal workout space in your home.

Most home workout areas tend to be located in attics, dens, or basements. Keep in mind that these places tend to be either quite dusty or damp. Exposure to increased amounts of dust mites or indoor mold in these areas might trigger allergic or asthma symptoms in susceptible people who are otherwise asymptomatic in the main living areas of their home. With some special adjustments you can still make your workout space relatively allergen-free. For dust allergies, remove carpeting and heavy drapes, which harbor dust mites. Clean the floor and equipment with a damp cloth at least once a week. If your allergy symptoms are moderately severe, you may want to invest in a quality air filter to remove dust particles from the air. If your workout area is damp and musty, consider using a dehumidifier and wipe washable surfaces with a bleach-containing solution to remove mildew buildup at least once a month. If needed, consider employing a space heater in cooler areas to avoid a possible cold trigger for bronchospasm. Also, avoid using cleaning supplies with heavy fragrances; they may provoke wheezing in some atopic individuals.

Training outside the home and joining a health club also has its benefits. Some people need the motivation of getting out of the house and working out with other people. Health clubs usually provide a wide variety of equipment, free weights, and resistance machines as well as cardiovascular equipment. Many facilities offer classes, such as aerobics or spinning, and may have a swimming pool, sauna, basketball courts, and other amenities. The primary disadvantages are transportation and cost, which may be quite high for some clubs. Nevertheless, low-cost options may exist in your area. Many cities and towns have fitness facilities located in park district field houses, municipal centers, and community centers. Often they are less expensive than private health clubs but have many of the same offerings and provide a fun, safe atmosphere for working out. While you tour the club, make note of the cleanliness and amount of dust, which may be important factors if you have indoor allergies.

If you are in doubt about a certain facility, ask whether they offer a trial membership. Some clubs don't offer the opportunity to try out the facility for free, but most do allow you to purchase a 1-day pass, which is still a valuable option to see whether the place suits your needs and likes. When you are investing your valuable time and money into a workout facility, it is important to ensure it meets your individual requirements.

More on Allergies and Asthma in the Weight Room

In general, allergic disease shouldn't interfere with weight training. As discussed in other chapters of this book, most asthma and urticaria (hives) are triggered by more aerobic activities. Allergic rhinitis is often triggered by outdoor allergens, which are unlikely to affect your strength training routine unless you are working out on Venice Beach! Nevertheless, people with allergic conditions need to keep in mind some important tips so that their allergies do not interfere with their strength training.

First of all, many people with allergic rhinitis or asthma take medications to control their symptoms. Many medications, especially antihistamines, have side effects that may potentially interfere with working out with weights. Many antihistamines, especially first-generation H2 blockers such as diphenhydramine, may cause drowsiness and fatigue in some people. These individuals might consider taking their medications after their strength training session, if possible, to avoid somnolence during the workout.

If you have EIA and have included cardiovascular training in your strength training routine, you may require self-administration of albuterol or another bronchodilator before using the treadmill or elliptical trainer. On the other hand, if using a bronchodilator makes you jittery, you may want to forgo weight training on those days after using your inhaler. Knowing your triggers and how the medication affects you is the key to avoiding problems.

Probably the most important factor to keep in mind is the environment in which you will be training. One of the most common allergens is dust (mites), and training indoors may be difficult for some people with severe dust allergies. If the room, either at home or at the fitness facility, is dusty, you may need to take medication, such as an antihistamine, before working out. If medication is necessary, a steroid nasal spray or a newer second-generation antihistamine can help avoid drowsiness. If you have asthma symptoms triggered by dust allergy, you should discuss

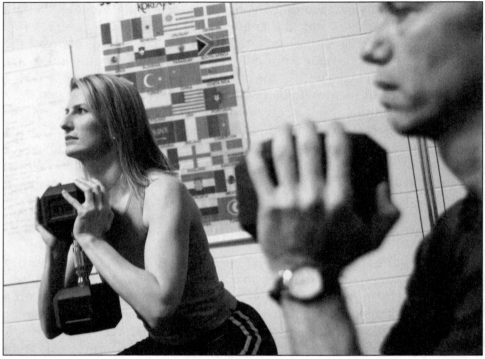

To ensure the best possible strength training experience, make sure your training environment is clean and doesn't contain symptom triggers, such as mold and dust mites.

with your physician whether you might require a controller medication such as an inhaled corticosteroid or a leukotriene modifier to decrease your susceptibility to respiratory complications of working out in a dusty environment. At the very least, consider using a bronchodilator approximately 10 to 15 minutes before working out. Unfortunately, most weight rooms can be quite dusty and thus may negatively impact your workout. Nevertheless, either searching out a clean gym or using medications as described will likely allow you to strength train successfully.

Recommended Strength Exercises

You can develop a balanced resistance training program with a few basic exercises. Your routine should include exercises for the upper and lower body and work opposing muscle groups around major joints. Try to dedicate equal time to all muscle groups for a symmetrical look and to avoid the problems associated with joint imbalance. Whether your goal is improved strength for sports or simply toning up for activities of daily living, I recommend focusing on your core muscle groups. These muscles include the chest, shoulders, back, abdominals, and pelvic stabilizers. We use the core muscle groups in almost every activity and sport; maintaining core strength is the key to maintaining functionality.

Before attempting these exercises, remember to review the guidelines mentioned earlier. Also, keep in mind the following:

- Maintain proper form and technique.
- Control the weight through the entire range of motion.
- Breathe in and out appropriately, and do not hold your breath.
- Keep your spine in neutral position, avoiding arching your back or slouching.
- For standing exercises, keep your knees and hips slightly bent.

Upper Body Exercises

Several basic exercises exist for the core muscles of the upper body. You should start with the basic bench press for chest, latissimus pull-down, reverse fly, and row for back as well as abdominal and trunk stabilizing exercises. Also included are some basic strength building exercises for the arms and hands.

CHEST FLY

This exercise helps define the central portion of the chest. Lying on your back, grasp a light weight in each hand and, with your elbows bent, lower the weights to your sides at chest level. As you exhale, slowly raise the weights until they meet above and out in front of your chest. The motion of squeezing the weights together works the inner chest. Slowly lower the weights to the starting position, then repeat.

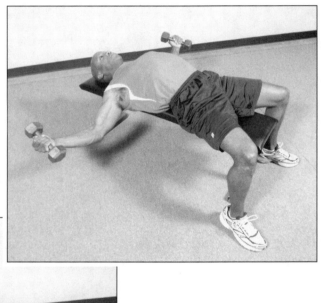

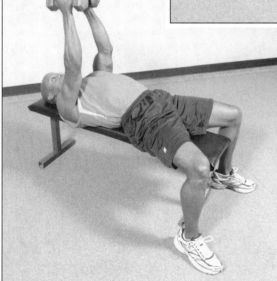

CHEST PRESS

The chest press is ideal for the large pectoralis major muscle but also activates some triceps fibers as well. Most weightlifters depend on the bench press to increase the overall size of their chest. For exercisers who don't have the same goal, perform the bench press with free weights (dumbbells) rather than with a barbell. Stabilizing each dumbbell through the range of motion requires you to activate many accessory fibers within the pectoralis muscle itself and thus provides a better workout. The traditional barbell bench press can be unsafe, especially for teens. Serious injury or death can result if the weight is too heavy and the barbell comes crashing down on your head, neck, chest, or abdomen. If you are still determined to perform a bench press with a barbell, at least use a spotter to help ensure safety.

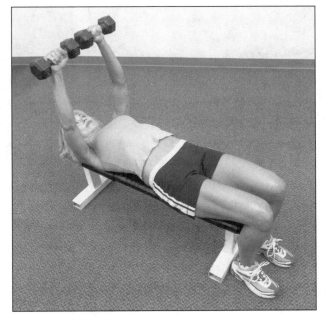

To perform a dumbbell bench press, lie on a bench with your feet flat and your knees bent at 90 degrees. With your weights in both hands, arms out to your sides, and elbows bent to 90 degrees, exhale and slowly lift the weights straight toward the ceiling, bringing the weights together. Hold for a second, then slowly lower the weight back to the starting position while inhaling, and then repeat. If you use rubber tubing or a pulley machine, be sure it is long enough to go under your shoulders as you lie on top of it—the motion is otherwise the same as with free weights.

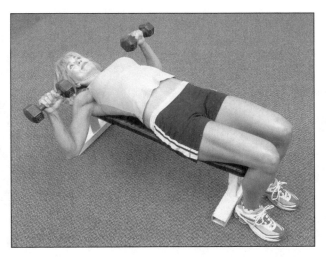

LATISSIMUS PULL-DOWN

The latissimus (lat) pull-down is a great exercise for your upper back, or latissimus dorsi muscles, but it also works your biceps and chest. Sitting for this exercise helps you stabilize the weight, so usually it is done with a pulley machine at the gym. Nevertheless, you can also do the lat pull-down with tubing at home by attaching the tubing to the top of a door. If you are doing this exercise on the machine, remember to pull the weight to the front (the top of your chest) and not to the back. Pulling the weight down behind the shoulder places a large unbalanced load on your rotator cuff and may cause shoulder problems.

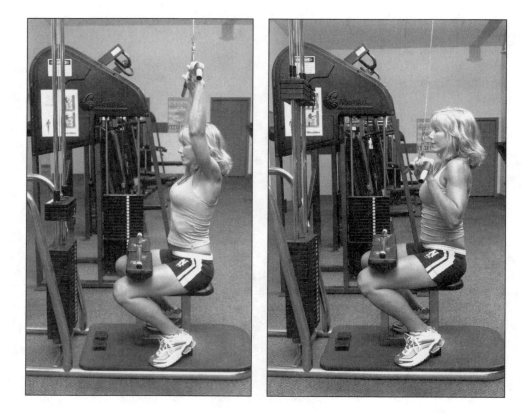

REVERSE FLY

The reverse fly is often commonly referred to as a bent-over lateral raise. The reverse fly works the posterior deltoid, the large superficial muscle of the shoulder, as well as some trapezius and rhomboid fibers. Choose a light weight in each hand, and bend over at the waist with your knees bent slightly. Keeping your back straight during the exercise is important to avoid low-back strain. With the weights initially hanging down in front of you, slowly lift them out to the sides and hold briefly. Avoid locking your elbows. Slowly return the weights to the initial position, then repeat.

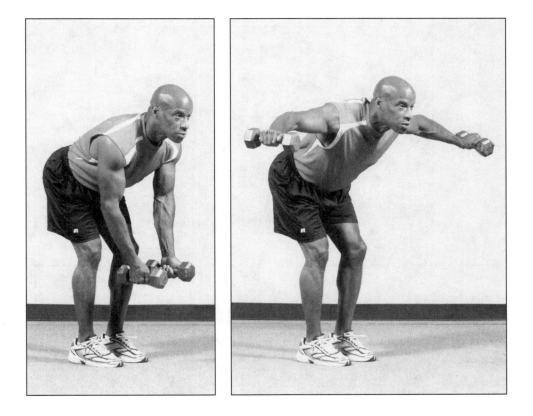

ROW

The row is another basic exercise for the back with a little more emphasis on the lower back. To perform this exercise on the row machine or with tubing, sit with your legs straight out in front of you. If you are using tubing, hook the loops around your feet and grasp the free ends. Pull the handles or the tubing ends toward you in a controlled fashion, bringing your hands to the sides near your chest. You can also perform this exercise with free weights in a bent-over row: Place one knee on a bench and the other on the floor, and bend over so that your back is parallel to the floor. With a weight in one hand hanging in front of (and below) you, slowly lift the weight until it reaches your hip, then return it to the starting position. Make sure to keep your back straight during the exercise.

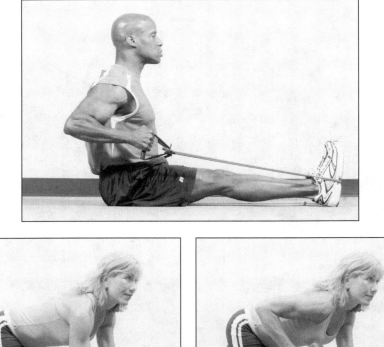

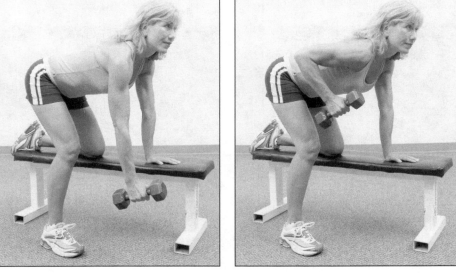

BICEPS CURL

Sitting or standing, the key to the biceps curl is strict form. Start with free weights or tubing in each hand, palms facing up. Slowly bend your elbow, lifting the weight toward your shoulder, hold briefly, and then slowly lower the weight again. Do not lock your elbows at the starting and stopping position; keep them slightly bent. Maintain correct form by keeping your arms at the sides. Avoid moving your elbows out to the sides or swinging them with each repetition.

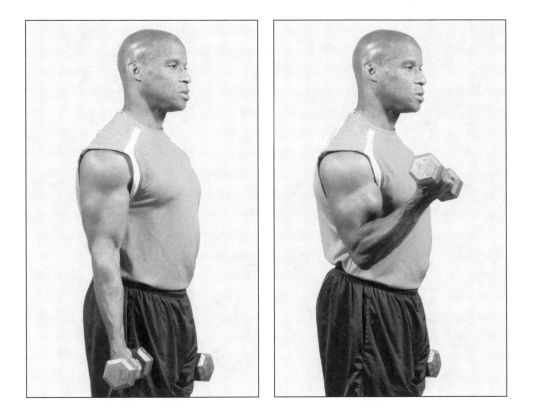

TRICEPS CURL

You can do the triceps curl with tubing or with free weights one arm at a time, although the triceps press machine allows you to train both arms at the same time. Sit or stand. Grasp the weight in your hand, and place it behind your head. Starting with your elbow bent, slowly lift the weight by straightening your elbow so that the finished position is above your head. You will notice the triceps completely contracted at that stage. Slowly lower the weight to the starting position. After performing the desired number of repetitions with one arm, switch the weight to the other hand and repeat.

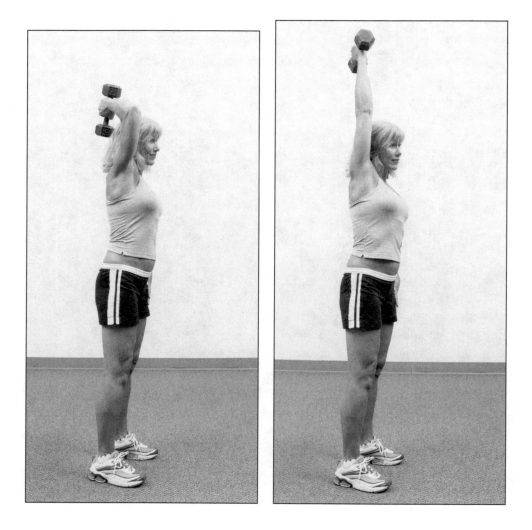

Abdominal and Low-Back Exercises

Most people with low-back pain do not realize that strengthening the abdominal muscles is imperative to maintaining a healthy, pain-free back. The basic crunch is a better exercise for your abdomen than the traditional sit-up, which places a lot of strain on your lower back. The oblique crunch works the side abdominals—the internal and external obliques.

Back stabilizing exercises also are important in eliminating low-back pain. Mechanical low-back pain is a common complaint in both active and nonactive individuals. Most back pain is actually related to overuse and muscle strain. Weak back and abdominal muscles lead to chronic low-back pain. By strengthening your back muscles, you will maintain better posture, have more trunk stability, and improve pain-free motion.

CAT-CAMEL

The cat-camel is a basic exercise for proper back maintenance. Start on your hands and knees with the back straight, and in a controlled fashion gently sag, then arch, your back. Repeat several times. Resist the temptation to hold your breath—it is important to slowly inhale and exhale during the exercise.

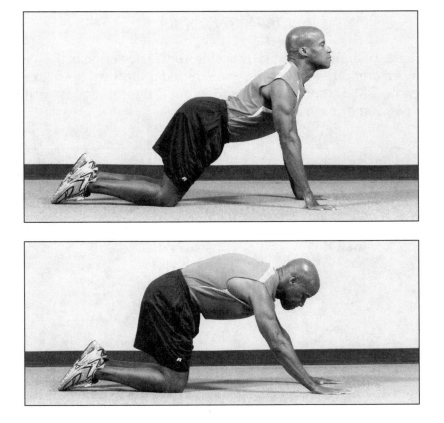

CRUNCH

For the crunch or curl-up, lie on your back with your knees bent and your feet flat. Slowly raise your shoulder blades off the ground, squeeze your abdominal muscles, and hold for a second. Lower your shoulders until they are flat on the ground, then repeat.

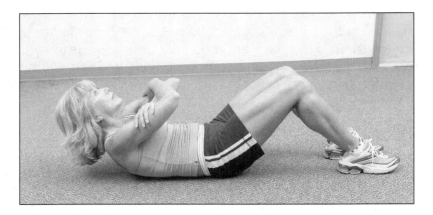

OBLIQUE CRUNCH

To work the oblique abdominal muscles, the basic action is the same but instead of symmetrically curling your shoulders toward both knees, aim for one knee. Make sure to alternate left and right obliques with either each repetition or each set.

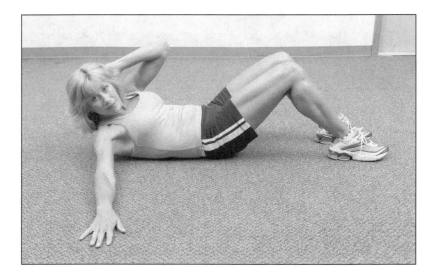

BIRD-DOG

The bird-dog stabilizes the spine, the gluteus maximus, hamstrings, and shoulder girdle muscles. Start on your hands and knees. Slowly push your left leg back and almost straighten it while simultaneously reaching your right arm straight out ahead of you. Hold for 10 to 15 seconds, then repeat with the left arm and right leg.

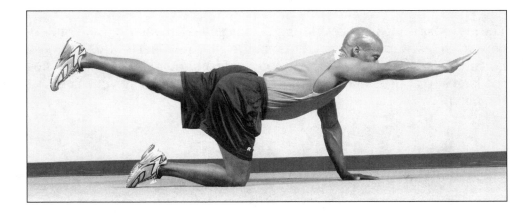

PLINTH

The plinth works your quadratus lumborum muscle to stabilize your spine. Start by lying on your side with your knees bent to 90 degrees. With your forearm on the ground and your elbow directly under your shoulder, slowly raise your trunk and hip off the ground. Hold for 10 to 15 seconds. Then slowly lower to the starting position and repeat. When you have finished, make sure to repeat the desired number of repetitions lying on the other side as well.

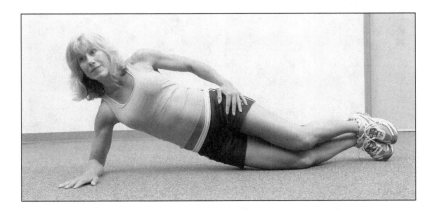

Lower Body Exercises

While upper body strength is obviously important for activities such as reaching and pulling, in addition to overhead throwing sports, lower body strength is important for mobilization and maintaining lower extremity joint function. Many of these exercises can be done using your own body weight or tubing as resistance.

LEG PRESS

The leg press is ideal for developing strong gluteal, hamstring, and quadriceps muscles. Resistance machines at the gym are ideal for this exercise. Be sure to maintain strict form. Keep the feet shoulder-width apart, flex the knees to approximately 90 degrees, and avoid locking your knees at the finish.

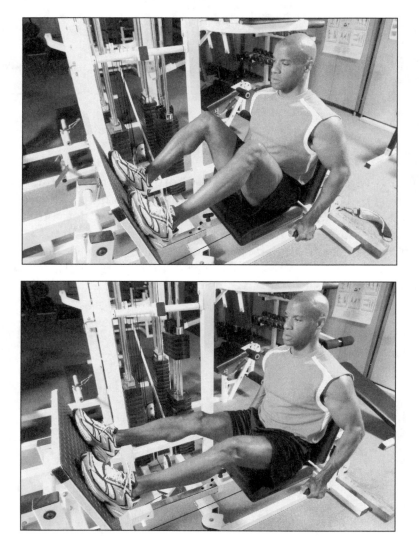

SQUAT

For squats, use light to moderate weight so as to lessen the low-back tension. Start in a standing position with your feet shoulder-width apart.

Bend your knees and hips slightly while keeping your low back straight, and then slowly stand up straight. Do not lock your knees at the finish. Slowly lower again, then repeat.

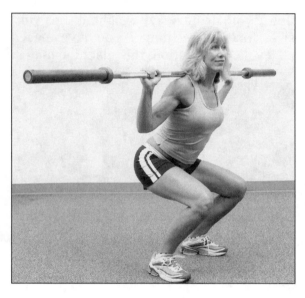

KNEE AND HIP EXTENSION AND FLEXION

The easiest way to make this exercise a closed-chain activity is to perform a lunge. Stand with your feet a few inches apart. Take a large step forward

with one foot, bending your knee until it almost touches the ground, then return to a standing position. Do the same with the other foot, and then repeat. To increase resistance you may hold light weights in your hands.

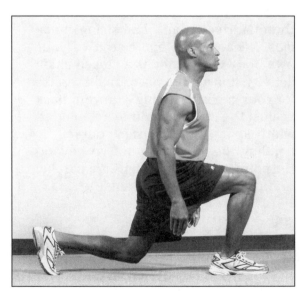

LEG EXTENSION

The leg extension machine is a gym standard and one that works well to develop the quadriceps muscles. Slowly raise the weight by extending your knees, pause briefly at the top, and slowly lower to the starting position. Avoid using heavy weight at the gym; this exercise can place a lot of stress on the knee joint. If you have kneecap pain, common in runners of all levels, use caution; this machine may increase your pain.

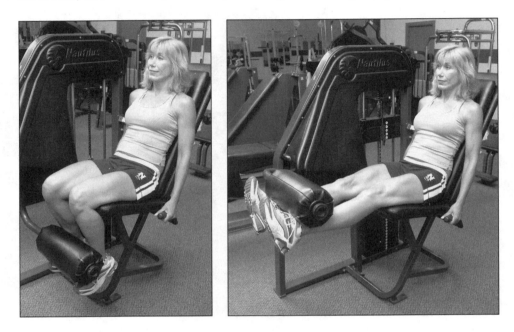

You may prefer the wall slide to work the quadriceps (and hamstring) muscles. Because this exercise uses your own body weight and is a closed-chain activity, it is a more functional exercise for your knees. Standing with your back against the wall and your feet shoulder-width apart, slowly lower yourself by bending the knees. Do not go beyond the point where your thighs are parallel to the floor (a 90-degree angle).

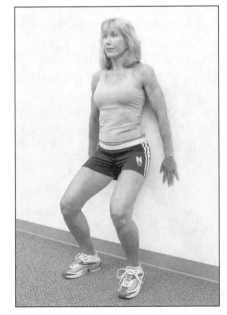

Sample Strength Programs

Tables 4.2, 4.3, and 4.4 provide a few sample strength training programs that you can use at home or at a gym. The initial program (table 4.2) starts with lower intensity and more repetitions. Exercisers with more experience can start at higher resistance (table 4.3 or 4.4). Remember that these samples are just that—samples of possible routines. They are not meant to be the last word on exercise. Feel free to adapt them as you need to, and, even if you do follow them initially, please expand on them later to liven up your routine.

Table 4.2 Initial Strength Program

Frequency	Intensity	Repetitions	Sets	Day 1	Day 2	Day 3
2-3 times/ week	50% of 1 RM	10-15	1-3	Chest press, biceps curl, triceps curl, push-up	Lat pull-down, row, hip extension, leg press, hamstring curl, hip abduction	Abdominals, cardiovascular

Table 4.3 Intermediate Strength Program

Frequency	Intensity	Repetitions	Sets	Day 1	Day 2	Day 3
3 times/ week	65% of 1 RM	10	3-4	Chest press, chest fly, triceps curl	Lat pull-down, row, standing biceps curl	Hip extension, leg press, hamstring curl, hip abduction, lunge

Table 4.4 Advanced Strength Program

Frequency	Intensity	Repetitions	Sets	Day 1	Day 2	Day 3
3-4 times/ week	80% of 1 RM	8-10	3-4	Chest press,* chest fly,* triceps curl	Lat pull-down, row, concentration biceps curl, standing biceps curl	Hip extension, leg press, hamstring curl, hip abduction/ adduction

*May be done with bench on incline or decline to work upper and lower chest.

Stretching and Functional Flexibility

Stretching exercises increase muscle-tendon unit flexibility. Flexibility is the ability to move a joint through its complete range of motion. Maintaining flexibility is important for several reasons. First, it facilitates joint movement, which is important for anyone who wants to stay active. Flexibility increases blood and nutrient supply to joints. The improved neuromuscular adaptation (the subconscious awareness of joint position in space) leads to improved balance and coordination. Stretching certain key muscle groups, such as the hamstrings, can improve the biomechanics around joints such as the knee and, as a result, decrease pain. Finally, flexibility is one of the key elements of the fitness triangle, allowing us to achieve greater strength and cardiorespiratory fitness. Flexibility depends on multiple factors, including distensibility of the joint capsule, adequate warm-up, muscle viscosity, and ligamentous and tendinous compliance. Some of these components are specific to the individual; others can be improved with practice and repetition. Flexibility is joint specific and, while no one test assesses total body flexibility, you can measure the flexibility of a given joint and therefore assess progress as you continue your workouts.

The body is multidimensional. Joints in the body move in multiple dimensions. Loss of motion in one plane will inhibit motion in the other two planes, thus creating abnormal motion and abnormal forces elsewhere in the body and ultimately leading to dysfunction. In other words, disuse or improper training of even certain muscle fibers within a muscle group can lead to abnormal stresses on the adjacent joint and result in dysfunction. A classic example is the knee. The quadriceps acts to extend the knee, and the medial component, the vastus medialis oblique (VMO), attaches medially to the kneecap and pulls it toward center (toward the other knee). Many athletes, however, fail to train the VMO; in fact, they often have atrophy, or wasting, of the VMO. These individuals usually also have tight hamstring muscles on the back of the knee, which can also affect the alignment of the kneecap in relation to the thighbone. This problem results in abnormal tracking of the kneecap, more irritation of the kneecap on the thighbone, and a condition known as patellofemoral stress syndrome, a common problem in young athletes. Strengthening the VMO component of the quadriceps and stretching the hamstring muscles will help better align the kneecap, biomechanically change the forces acting on the knee joint, and decrease anterior knee pain over time.

Stretching is the action we use to achieve flexibility. The benefits of stretching, therefore, include decreased muscle stiffness, less muscle soreness, and increased flexibility. Certain types of stretching may improve performance and help prevent injuries. Many types of stretching exist, but to discuss all in depth would require another entire book.

The three primary types of stretching exercises are static, ballistic, and proprioceptive neuromuscular facilitation (PNF). Static exercises slowly stretch a tendon, hold it in the stretched state for a period of time, and then return it to its resting length. ACSM recommends holding static stretches for 10 to 30 seconds (Lloyd 2001). Ballistic stretching involves repetitive bouncing movements that rapidly stretch and then relax the muscle-tendon unit. In PNF stretching, the muscle-tendon units are alternately contracted isometrically and then stretched passively. ACSM recommends holding the contraction for 6 seconds, then performing an assisted stretch for 10 to 30 seconds. Many PNF techniques exist, but most require an experienced trainer or therapist.

Traditionally stretching has been primarily static and uniplanar. Traditional stretching is also time-consuming and limited to specific joints. Focusing on only static stretching leads to improper performance and may increase your risk for injury and therefore decrease your overall strength. Functional stretching, on the other hand, is dynamic, activity specific, fun, and effective. Functional stretching uses multiple joints in three dimensions and results in better compliance. If you are trying to decide on which type of stretching to incorporate into your workout, functional stretching is the way to go.

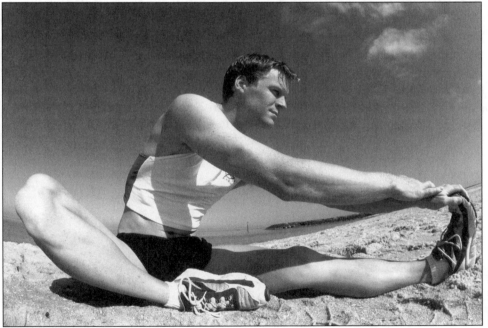

© Sport the Library

Stretching supplements the other two parts of a comprehensive exercise program—strength training and aerobic exercise—and it also helps prevent injuries.

So, what is functional stretching? Functional stretching involves stretching and moving a joint through a multiplanar range of motion rather than just stretching and holding in one position. As an example consider the hamstring stretch. With the classic static stretch, you place the foot on an elevated surface such as a step, bend at the waist, and lean into the stretch, holding for 30 seconds and then relaxing. With a dynamic hamstring stretch, you lean toward the foot and hold, but then you move the trunk from side to side, adding an extra twist to the classic stretch. In this manner the stretch is expanded to three dimensions, working the hamstring in three planes and simulating the way the muscle works in real-life situations.

The timing of the stretch is also important. If you stretch before warming up, strength may be compromised. If you stretch after warming up, benefits include reduced delayed onset muscle soreness, improved stretch tolerance, and increased range of motion. Your stretch should follow your warm-up but precede your workout and place your joints through a full range of motion that simulates your actual anticipated exercise. In this manner you can precondition the muscles to the exercise you are going to perform and thus maximize your results.

ACSM recommends including stretching and flexibility exercises into a complete fitness routine (Lloyd 2001). A general stretching program should exercise the major muscle-tendon groups (e.g., quadriceps, gluteals/hamstrings/calves, shoulder girdle) and should include static, ballistic, or modified PNF techniques. Most experts now believe that stretching should be dynamic as well to imitate closely the same movements one uses in daily life. Focus on at least 4 repetitions for each muscle group and stretch at least 2 days a week. Remember to stretch to the point of slight discomfort but not to the point of pain. Stretching should not be painful. Also, inhale and exhale slowly during each stretch; holding your breath can be dangerous (see Valsalva Maneuver on page 114).

Recommended Stretches

Many of these stretches are static exercises. They are easiest to explain but also quite effective. Included are some ideas for how to make these exercises more functional and dynamic.

NECK

Rotate your neck through an entire range of motion (forward flexion, lateral rotation and lateral bending, extension backward). Then practice neck glides. Keeping your chin level, glide your head straight back (as if you were giving yourself a double chin). Hold for 5 seconds. Repeat.

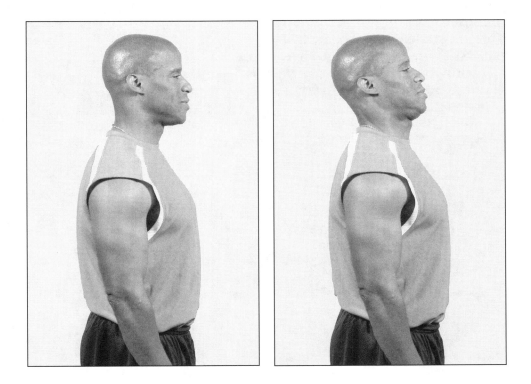

ARMS

For triceps, place your right hand behind your head and reach toward your left shoulder blade. Take your left hand and push your right elbow back to maximize the stretch on your right triceps. Hold 10 seconds, then repeat with the opposite arm.

To stretch your wrist extensors and flexors, hold one arm out in front of you. For your extensors, face one palm down toward your body flexed at the wrist, and with the other hand gently press the flexed hand toward you. Count to 10. Then, to stretch your flexors, face your palm away from your body, fingers up, and with your other hand gently press your extended hand toward you. Again, count to 10.

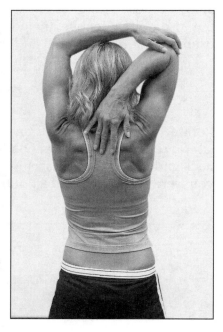

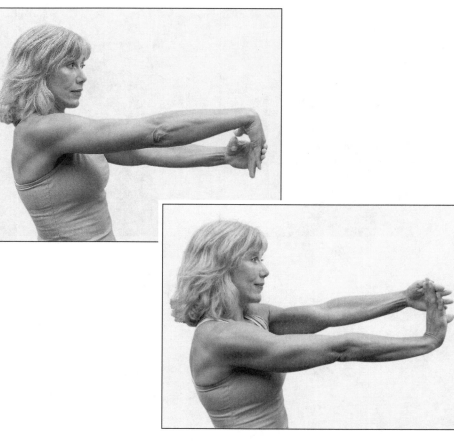

BACK

To stretch your upper back, reach out in front of you with both hands, arms straight, and grasp the hands together. Relax, and feel the stretch between your shoulder blades. Hold for 10 seconds.

To relax your low back, lie on the ground face up with the arms extended out to the sides, palms down. Slowly drop both knees to one side while turning your head to the opposite side. Keep your shoulders flat on the floor. Hold for 10 seconds. Return to the starting position, and repeat on the other side.

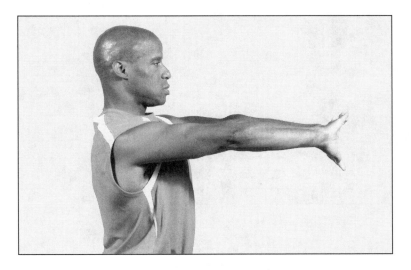

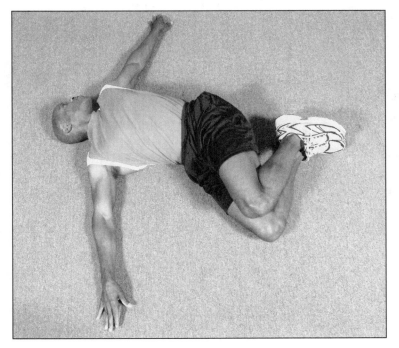

QUADRICEPS

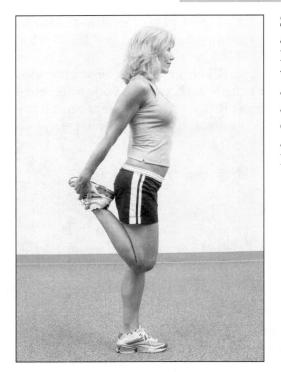

Standing, flex one knee maximally and grab your foot behind you. Pull the foot up toward your gluteals to maximally stretch your anterior thigh muscles. Hold for at least 10 seconds. To add in a dynamic twist, alternately flex and extend at the hip while still holding your foot.

GLUTEALS AND HAMSTRINGS

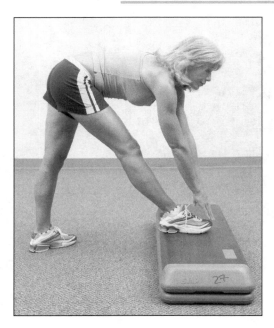

Standing, raise one foot and place it on a step. Keep the knee of the raised leg straight. Lean forward, reaching toward the toes of your raised foot. As you reach maximum forward flexion, hold this position for at least 10 seconds. To make this stretch dynamic, sway your body from side to side while leaning forward.

CALVES

Face a wall standing 2 feet away. Step forward with one foot, and keep this forward knee bent but the back knee straight. Lean forward as if doing a push-up, keeping both heels on the ground. Feel the stretch along your calves. Hold at least 10 seconds, then relax. Repeat with the other foot forward. To make this stretch more dynamic, repeat it with the back knee slightly bent.

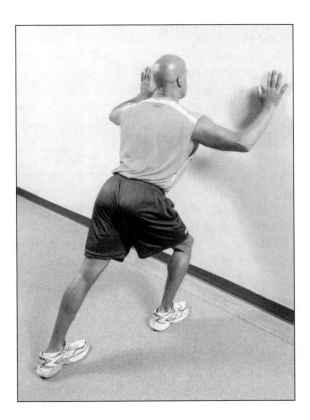

Safety Considerations

Like most sports and physical activities, strength training can bring some risks. Most are dangers resulting from poor form, improper training, or lack of spotting. You also need to exercise caution when stretching to avoid injuries from overstretching or improper technique. To minimize risks to personal safety, you may need to take precautions such as those mentioned throughout this chapter for people with respiratory symptoms related to allergies or asthma. Following are some basic, useful safety tips to keep in mind when strength training or stretching.

Valsalva Maneuver   Many people attempt to hold the breath when lifting heavy weight to generate more force. The problem with this is that exhaling against a closed glottis (windpipe) leads to increased pressure in the chest cavity, reducing venous blood flow to the heart. It also temporarily causes a rapid rise in blood pressure followed by a rapid fall in arterial blood pressure. It can make you feel dizzy and lightheaded, have blurred vision, and even pass out.

To avoid this situation, breathe properly during weightlifting. When applying the force against resistance, such as when pushing the weights up in a bench press, you should exhale. Inhale when lowering the weight and preparing for the next push. You should still be able to generate sufficient force to successfully complete the exercise and will avoid a potentially serious outcome. Breathing correctly is important not only for weight training but for aerobic exercise and stretching as well.

Common Cold   The common cold is not necessarily a reason to avoid exercise. While you should never exercise when you really do not feel well, you are unlikely to encounter any danger by exerting yourself when you have the sniffles. People with asthma should exercise caution when they have a cold; viral respiratory infections can trigger bronchospasm. Nevertheless, most athletes with asthma can still exercise regularly when they have a cold. In general, strength training is less likely to trigger bronchospasm than aerobic exercise; however, you still need to use caution in allergenic environments or when doing prolonged exercise routines (such as aerobic exercise and strength training during the same prolonged session).

Fever   Fever, however, is a different matter. A rise in core body temperature increases your risk of heat illness and dehydration. Fever is also nature's way of telling your body you need rest. You should never exercise if you have a fever or chills. Give your body a break, and when you recover you can hit the weights extra hard!

Eczema   Along with allergic rhinitis and asthma, eczema, or atopic dermatitis, makes up the trio called atopy, or atopic disease. With eczema the skin barrier is broken, which can increase the risk for skin infections. If you have eczema, you should ensure that the benches in the gym are wiped clean prior to use, wear water shoes on tiled floors, and avoid sharing towels. Also, use emollients liberally to maintain moisture within the skin and prevent dermatitis flare-ups. For the most part, however, you will be able to participate in weight training without any problem.

Exercise-Induced Urticaria In general, individuals with this condition experience hives when engaging in vigorous aerobic exercise. An athlete who is predisposed to urticaria with exercise should use care when training in hot environments. Ambient heat makes the skin release histamine, which can exacerbate itching and hives. If you have this condition, you may want to avoid stuffy gyms in hot, humid weather or premedicate with an antihistamine before your workout.

Stretching Technique Maintaining proper form during stretching is also paramount in importance. During a flexibility session, focus on performing each stretch smoothly and gracefully. The movements should flow easily. Avoid bouncing or brisk movements and concentrate on relaxing your muscle tone. You also need to avoid overstretching. Holding a particular stretch for too long (more than 30 seconds) or beyond the normal range of motion for that particular joint may decrease the tensile strength of that muscle unit and could lead to injury.

Summary

This chapter has given you some ideas for planning your strength training routine and flexibility program. You have learned about setting your intensity level, advancing your workout by adding resistance, maintaining proper technique, and the type of exercises and stretches you should perform. Remember, though, that the most important aspect of developing a resistance training program is achieving the goals you chose at the beginning. We all have different starting places and different objectives with training. Choosing realistic, attainable goals is the key to success. Once you meet those goals you can take a minute, reassess where you are, and decide on new goals for the future. Then, shake up your workout—change the body parts you train on certain days, add in new exercises, or even modify the exercises themselves (change from a flat bench press to an incline press). Keeping your workout fresh will help you achieve your new objectives and avoid hitting a plateau. As you get more comfortable with strength training and flexibility exercises, you will get a feel for what works for you and how to keep yourself motivated to succeed.

Do not let your asthma or allergies prevent you from getting stronger and more flexible. Most people with even severe allergic disease can strength train safely and still achieve their desired results. You may need to make small adjustments, such as the timing of your medication or avoiding certain environmental factors, but you will still be able to enjoy the advantages of resistance training. In fact, the benefits your body receives from a strength training program, such as increased metabolic rate and improved body composition, will have lasting positive effects on your overall health for years, even decades, to come!

ACTION PLAN:
BUILDING STRENGTH AND FLEXIBILITY

☐ Set realistic, attainable goals.

☐ Include warm-up and cool-down times before and after your routine.

☐ Include functional, dynamic stretching after your warm-up.

☐ Follow your schedule and intensity as determined in this chapter and based on your goals.

☐ Work major muscle groups, agonists, and antagonists.

☐ Take the muscle through a full range of motion.

☐ Focus on eccentric, closed-chain exercises.

☐ Remember that proper technique is paramount!

☐ Breathe during the exercise—don't hold your breath.

☐ Rest 1 or 2 minutes between sets.

☐ Monitor your progress, make changes as necessary, and vary your routine to avoid plateaus.

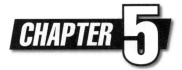

EXPLORING ALTERNATIVE FORMS OF EXERCISE

Matthew J. Brandon

With the growing interest in alternative medicine over the past two decades, new and timeless alternative remedies have come closer to the mainstream. Similar trends have occurred with exercise over the past two decades. Along with growing interest in traditional exercise programs, alternative modes of exercise have gained new heights of popularity in the health care, fitness, and rehabilitation fields. In my sports medicine practice, on any given day I may encounter the same number of patients taking yoga classes as patients playing softball. In fact, the exercise universe is becoming increasingly populated with participants in yoga, tai chi, Pilates, aerobics classes, stationary cycling classes, or aquatic exercise classes. I tend to divide the alternative modes of exercise into two categories: mind–body exercise programs and exercise programs adapted from more traditional exercise principles.

Yoga, tai chi, and Pilates can be grouped into mind–body alternative forms of exercise. The basic tenet of mind–body exercise is that emotion, thoughts, and behavior can affect your physiologic functions. Several psychophysical techniques exist; but yoga, tai chi, and Pilates are the most popular. Yoga and tai chi are the oldest and are steeped in Eastern tradition and philosophy. Pilates is a more Western method that is generally performed at a higher intensity. Each program allows participants to educate themselves about the body. The psyche controls the physical body. For example, emotional discord may lead to poor posture, muscle tension, and poor conditioning, and vice versa. These Eastern techniques focus on slow, purposeful movements with controlled, often deep breathing. An instructor guides the class through several purposeful movements with the participants concentrating on awareness of the body in space and time.

Scientific evidence shows that yoga improves pulmonary function. Yoga has been connected to improvements in asthma symptoms and exercise tolerance as well as improved mood and stress reduction. Vickers et al. (1997) reviewed the literature regarding yoga's positive effects on asthma and determined that the regulated breathing patterns practiced in yoga definitely reduced asthma symptom scores and improved exercise tolerance. Wolf et al. (1997) reviewed the scientific evidence regarding the benefits of tai chi. The review found that tai chi offers similar benefits but also improved balance, reducing falls among the elderly, and documented improvement in cardiovascular performance at all ages. Pilates has gained popularity for its improvement in core strength, movement efficiency, and flexibility. As you can see, it is no wonder these exercise classes have exploded in recent years. These classes may be a perfect fit for you, or you may consider an alternative form of a more traditional exercise program.

The rise in enrollment in aerobics classes and aquatic exercise classes is well established, but yoga, tai chi, stationary cycling, and Pilates classes are not trailing by much. I have family members, friends and patients who swear by the results of these programs. Regardless of the type of program you choose, you should check with your personal physician, physical therapist, or athletic trainer before taking an alternative exercise class.

These activities are usually performed in a class setting. My friends, family members, and patients find comfort and motivation from the class setting. They often tell me that exercising alone is boring but the classes bring more excitement and motivation. Class participants enjoy the benefit of encouragement from other participants and vice versa. Friends and couples are able to use fitness facilities and classes for socialization while reaping the benefits of exercise. Classes are often designed for individuals at the same fitness level and allay fears of embarrassment or being left behind.

People with asthma, EIA, or allergies may find other people in their classes with similar problems and find comfort in knowing they are not alone in their struggles. I have friends and patients who have been reminded by fellow classmates to take their inhaler or check their peak flow when they would have otherwise forgotten. I even have had a few friends discover they had EIA from observing classmates, and they subsequently consulted me about their condition. As stated previously, coughing, wheezing, breathlessness, extreme fatigue, and chest discomfort are all indications you may have asthma or EIA.

Selecting Activities That Fit Your Needs

Whether you have asthma, EIA, allergies, or any other condition, you should consider certain factors when choosing an alternative exercise class. The psychosocial benefits of group or class exercise are abundant, but the same situation may be detrimental if you choose the wrong class.

Table 5.1 outlines the 10 basic considerations when signing up for an exercise class. The most critical elements are the type of class, fitness level of class participants, and quality of the instructor. For people with asthma who have moderate control of symptoms and low fitness levels, a low-impact aerobic class or environmentally friendly aquatic exercise class would be a good adjunct to a traditional aerobic exercise program. Conversely, if you have aquagenic or cold urticaria, both physical allergies, an aquatic program may not be ideal. Spinning classes are ideal for fit individuals with asthma to maintain training effect when the weather calls for a change of environment. Perhaps you would like to combine aerobic fitness, balance, coordination, and strength training together in one exercise class. In that case, yoga and tai chi are probably the way to go.

Always choose a class at your fitness level. Ask whether you can try one class before signing up, and use the Karvonen formula or rating of

Table 5.1   Factors to Consider in Choosing an Exercise Class

Class fitness level	Enroll in the class that corresponds to your activity level: sedentary, mildly active, moderately active, active, or very active.
Instructor qualifications	Instructor is certified by an accredited agency and shows the ability to adapt to the needs and goals of the participants.
Class type	Exercise type should fit your goals and be within your capability.
Where and when	Choose a class you will be able to attend without difficulty.
Trial run	Test the class to determine whether it is suited to your needs.
Environment	Choose a class that is in an environment conducive to exercising with your allergic condition.
Special populations	You may choose a class specifically designed for people with asthma, EIA, or other allergies.
Facilities	Make sure the facilities have employees trained in basic CPR.
Cost	Explore all the costs and contracts involved; you may be locked into a class and instructor you do not like.
Flexibility	Make sure you can continue to participate in the class even if your allergic condition requires transient adjustments.

perceived exertion (RPE) scale (chapters 3 and 4) to assess the intensity level of the class. If choosing a class in which the activity is completely foreign, try starting at a lower intensity than you are accustomed to. You may ramp up your intensity at the next class based on your target heart rate, RPE, and asthma or EIA status.

You will respond differently to different instructors; stick with the instructor who provides a safe, stimulating, and enjoyable exercise class. Look into the instructor's qualifications, such as certifications from accredited agencies (e.g., the American Council on Exercise and the American College of Sports Medicine). Remember, a poor choice in exercise class can result in frustration, boredom, and even exacerbation of your asthma or allergies.

Each alternative exercise form has different but largely beneficial effects on health and fitness. Each form differs in its relation to asthma, EIA, and allergy. Some alternative exercise classes clearly benefit asthma and EIA while other classes have less scientific support. I strongly encourage you to use these forms of exercise as adjuncts to traditional aerobic exercise in the setting of asthma and EIA. Although accumulating evidence of health benefits is being discovered, the scientific base of evidence behind these alternative forms is much less than traditional exercise. You can rest assured that your allergic rhinitis or physical allergies, if treated properly, should not interfere or prevent experimentation with alternative forms of exercise. Explore these exercise programs and classes, but keep in mind that they are not replacements for traditional exercises.

Yoga

Yoga has been practiced for centuries in mainly Eastern cultures. The goal of yoga is to liberate the discord between the mind and body through various movements and breathing techniques. Hatha yoga is a practice that has been well studied in its relation to asthma, EIA, and other pulmonary conditions. Hatha yoga incorporates techniques that involve postures, actions, and relaxation to improve posture, balance, flexibility, strength, and physical conditioning. If you are considering yoga for conditioning, you should concentrate on hatha yoga and patterned breathing to improve your asthma and EIA symptoms. Specific techniques, called pranayamas, involve controlled, deep inspiration; suspension of the breath; and slow, controlled exhalation. Naturally, the respiratory muscles are conditioned and strengthened. Patterned deep breathing has been part of pulmonary rehabilitation, so you can see how hatha yoga would be beneficial for your asthma or EIA. Asanas are the techniques that involve holding different postures to allow the mind to be aware of the body in space and time. Holding postures will serve to improve balance, muscular strength, flexibility, and coordination. Together asanas and pranayamas serve to improve pulmonary performance with exercise. Hatha yoga can involve

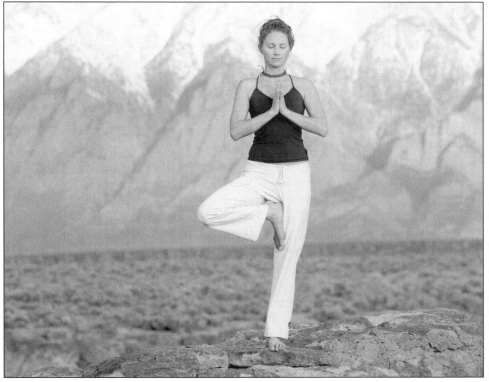

Hatha yoga and patterned breathing techniques help control asthma and allergy symptoms by conditioning and strengthening the respiratory muscles.

several other techniques beyond the scope of this chapter. Hatha yoga is a great way to augment your traditional aerobic exercise and incorporate strength and flexibility training in one activity.

Many scientists have studied the benefits of yoga. Joshi et al. (1992), Makwana et al. (1988), Rai and Ram (1993), Telles et al. (2000), Bera and Rajapurkar (1993), Raju et al. (1997), Ray et al. (2001), and Tran et al. (2001) are examples of studies boasting yoga's benefits on pulmonary function. The findings are summarized next. Some of these studies have been under scrutiny for their methods, but no study has shown that yoga worsens asthma, EIA, or allergic conditions. The majority of studies are published in the Indian medical literature. However, studies on the effects of yoga have been published in several well-respected Western medical journals. In the late 1980s and early 1990s many studies demonstrated an increase in FEV 1 (forced expiratory volume in 1 second) and peak flow rates in healthy male subjects. As stated in previous chapters, these measurements are predictors of performance in asthma and EIA. Additional studies as recent as 2000 and 2001 showed similar improvements in FEV 1 and peak flow of female subjects participating in yoga. You may wonder whether these studies show evidence that yoga will reduce your coughing, wheezing, and breathlessness with exercise. They do not, but others have shown the results you are asking about. In 1985, 1986, and 1990 scientific evaluations of hatha yoga showed improvements in FEV 1 and peak flow of people with mild to moderate asthma. Seventy percent of the subjects of these studies were able to decrease the frequency of rescue inhaler use and experienced less wheezing, coughing, and breathlessness with other physical activity. Similar studies in 2000 and 2001 showed improvement in breathing and tolerance of exercise but failed to produce improvements in lung function measurements such as FEV 1 and peak flow. Conflicting studies do exist. Sabina et al. (2005) studied yoga intervention in the treatment of mild to moderate asthma and determined no benefit of yoga on pulmonary function in asthma or EIA. These studies did not focus on hatha yoga.

Choosing a yoga class requires attention to many details for assurance of a safe and beneficial experience. No specific contraindications to yoga participation exist if you have asthma, EIA, or allergies. As with any new exercise program, make sure your peak flow is greater than 80 percent of predicted value and you are not experiencing asthma or allergy symptoms. Premedicating with two puffs of your rescue inhaler 10 to 15 minutes before the session is always a good idea. Adhering to a sound treatment regimen for allergic rhinitis is paramount for participating in a yoga class. Keeping the nasal passages clear should allow for better breathing. Hatha yoga is preferred to improve your pulmonary function, but any yoga program involving controlled breathing techniques may help. Be certain that your class is a beginner class starting with basic postures with gradual inclusion of more complicated postures or even actions. The optimal class duration is 40 to 60 minutes, excluding appropriate warm-up and cool-down. The actual class time may be up to 90 minutes. Know your yoga instructor. Inquire about the instructor's experience (usually more experienced instructors are better), and check with the Yoga Alliance Registry. Take steps to make your instructor aware of your needs and medical conditions. Optimize your class environment by choosing indoor, climate-controlled classes or outdoor classes in favorable weather, pollution, or pollen-count days (see chapter 7). I recommend comfortable, loose clothing with room for your medications and rescue inhaler.

Tai Chi

The practice of tai chi has been popular in China and other Eastern countries for hundreds of years. Originating from the martial arts, tai chi in literal translation means "the grand ultimate fist." The popularity of tai chi has risen dramatically in Western countries over the last few decades. Tai chi exercise improves blood pressure, aerobic endurance, and respiratory function. This form of mind–body exercise allows participants to concentrate on breathing while performing slow, controlled movements. Tai chi,

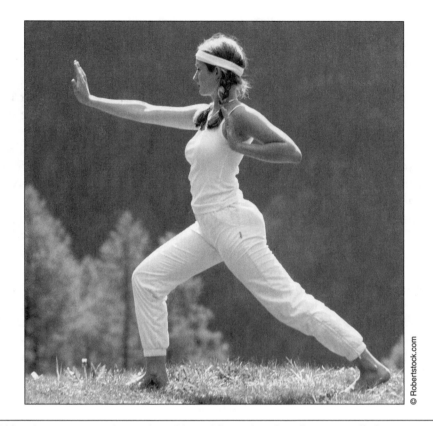

Tai chi involves concentration on breathing while performing slow, controlled movements.

like yoga, has many styles incorporating 100 or more movements for each style. The different styles of tai chi allow you to choose the style that fits your goals and current fitness level. Tai chi exercise employs asymmetric extremity movements, weight shifting, trunk rotation, and holding erect head and neck positions. Changing posture height changes the intensity of the workout. I am not aware of any specific warning or contraindication regarding tai chi exercise and asthma, EIA, or allergy.

The lion's share of medical literature involving tai chi and lung function is limited by small sample sizes and poor study design. Further, very little evidence exists about the effect of tai chi on asthma, EIA, and allergy. Several studies have shown improvements in aerobic exercise capacity and lung function of subjects participating in tai chi exercise. Similar to studies of traditional exercise, tai chi studies have shown different results based on intensity, duration, and frequency of exercise. The greatest benefits of tai chi exercise seem to occur with the more intense styles of tai chi. Also, the most sedentary individuals seem to demonstrate the greatest benefit. The flexibility of tai chi with its varying styles may explain why adherence to tai chi exercise programs is good.

Before starting a tai chi exercise class, make sure your asthma and EIA are under good control. Certain styles of tai chi can produce exercise intensities of 40 to 60 percent of maximal heart rate. If you are experiencing coughing, wheezing, chest discomfort, or breathlessness, check with your personal physician before starting a tai chi class. Make sure your peak flow is greater than 80 percent of your predicted value, and premedicate with your rescue inhaler. Ask the instructor about his or her qualifications and experience. A good starting point may be with a home exercise video from a reputable source. You should start out with shorter (20- to 30-minute) sessions involving higher positions and the minimum number of postures. If your activity level is low, a class focusing on high squat positions would be ideal. The Yang style of tai chi involves up to 108 different postures and uses low squat positions to maximize the intensity of the exercise session. Your beginning intensity level may rest somewhere between the two positions. Any tai chi class should last no more than 60 minutes, including an appropriate warm-up and cooldown. Consult with your instructor to adapt the positions and postures to your desired intensity level. Wear loose, comfortable clothing, keep your rescue inhaler handy, and always choose an optimal environment for your exercise class. If your tai chi class is held outdoors and you experience allergic symptoms, adhering to the guidelines in chapter 7 will optimize your exercise environment and enhance your enjoyment of the session.

Pilates

Joseph H. Pilates, born in Germany, developed an exercise form based on Eastern and Western exercise philosophies. Pilates' new exercise form emphasized the mind–body concept and was initially known as *contrology*. Pilates moved to New York City and opened a studio in 1926. Pilates, which the exercise form is now named, was very popular among athletes and especially dancers. Dancers swore the exercise method kept them injury free and, when injured, returned them to the performance stage quicker. Pilates programs vary from instructor to instructor. An important distinction exists between traditional Pilates and Pilates-based instruction. Traditional Pilates training involves a series of exercises with minimal movement and few repetitions. Traditionalists also use very few apparatus or equipment. Generally, the program is either performed as a series of mat exercises (using a mat on the floor) or exercises on the chosen apparatus. Pilates-based instruction may incorporate some Pilates principles but may incorporate other exercises and equipment as well.

Pilates exercise concentrates on your core muscle strength, or "powerhouse," using the Pilates nomenclature. Your core muscles include the pelvic, abdominal, and back muscles. The exercise program focuses on stabilizing the trunk through use of abdominal, pelvic, and spinal muscles in varying movement patterns. Coordination, flexibility, muscle strength, joint range of motion, and postural improvements are all benefits associ-

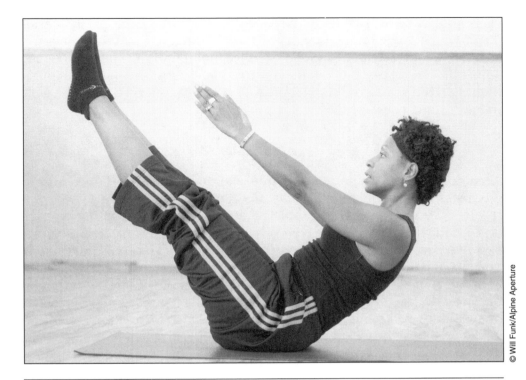

Pilates is great for working the core muscles and improving coordination, flexibility, and strength; just make sure it is done in addition to aerobic exercise, not in place of it, for better allergy and asthma help.

ated with Pilates exercise. Regulated breathing patterns during Pilates exercise help improve endurance. Little scientific evidence exists to substantiate these claims, but overwhelming popular support does exist for this exercise form. Measurements of exercise intensity have shown that beginning, moderate, and advanced Pilates exercise sessions were equal to low-moderate, moderate, and high-moderate intensity level traditional exercise, respectively. At present no definite proven benefit or contraindication exists of Pilates with regard to asthma or EIA.

Before starting a Pilates class, you need to determine the intensity level of the class. Ask the instructor at what level the class is set, and then give the class a trial run. Try using the RPE scale to determine whether the class is appropriate for your fitness level. Assessing the severity of your asthma by symptoms and peak flow is also very important. Seek medical attention if you are concerned about your asthma or EIA. Using your allergy medications and optimizing the environment will help keep your nasal passages open for optimal regulated breathing. If you are sedentary, a less-intense Pilates class is recommended. Check www.pilatesmethodalliance. org to search for certified Pilates trainers and other information. Instructors are considered experienced if they have 3 to 5 years of instruction under their belt with other continuing education activities. Your Pilates class should be at least 30 minutes in duration with appropriate warm-up and cool-down. Remember, if you have asthma or EIA, Pilates is not a substitute for traditional aerobic exercise, but it certainly is an excellent adjunct form of exercise. If you participate in weight training, you can do Pilates on the same day, but include a 24-hour rest period before the next weight-training session.

Aerobics

Aerobics refers to a series of group exercises that use large muscle groups in a rhythmic, repetitive nature. Aerobics classes are a good way to diversify your existing aerobic or strength training routine or may be a good whole-body, primary exercise program. Aerobics classes can improve aerobic exercise capacity. Aerobics also claims cardiovascular benefits and improvements in pulmonary function. Aerobics classes may improve your asthma symptoms and tolerance to other aerobic activities but provide less of a benefit than traditional walking, running, cycling, or swimming programs. Traditional programs also boast more scientific evidence backing their benefit claims. Aerobics classes differ greatly in their design. Classes may be classified by environment (land or aquatic). Other classifications may be based on type of activity, level of intensity (high or low impact), and emphasis on a specific conditioning principle. For example, stationary cycling classes (sometimes referred to as Spinning) tend to emphasize aerobic endurance as opposed to muscle strength and vary in intensity depending on speed and amount of time out of the saddle. Participants enjoy the social interaction and fun environment of these classes. Most classes incorporate music, and classmates are encouraged to interact with the instructor and each other. Because so many choices exist, you really need to look at your current fitness level and fitness goals to decide on the right class for you.

Know your current fitness level before signing up for a class. If you are sedentary to moderately active, you should choose a class of low to moderate intensity and shorter duration. For example, a low-impact step aerobics class of 20 to 30 minutes in duration may be ideal if you are sedentary. High-impact classes involve hopping and jumping. Low-impact classes involve always keeping one foot on the ground. Also, changing the height of a step will increase the intensity. Low- and high-impact aerobics intensities are comparable to walking or running, and you may view a changing step height or addition of weights similar to adding hills to a walking or running program. Try a test run of each class to determine your percentage of target heart rate or RPE. I recommend starting at 50 percent of your target heart rate or light to moderate perceived exertion (see chapter 3 for specific details). I do not recommend starting above 70 percent of your target heart rate with any new exercise class even if you are already fit and very active. If you are a beginner, you might want to

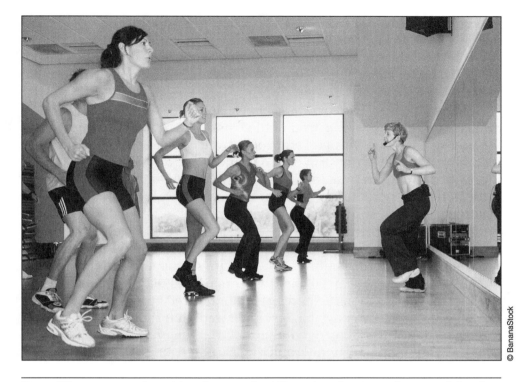

Many different types of aerobics classes exist. When choosing one, take note of the class environment and make sure the instructor knows of your asthma or allergies.

look for classes such as low-impact aerobics, water aerobics, or easy step aerobics. If you're looking for higher-intensity classes, look for high-impact classes, power step classes, and boxing aerobics. If your asthma or EIA flares, drop the level of intensity by returning to a lower-impact class or you may alter other class conditions. When your symptoms and peak flow return to normal, you may return to the previous level of intensity.

Water aerobics provides an optimal exercise environment for asthma, EIA, and allergy sufferers. Water aerobics certainly reduces the chances for bronchospasm or asthma attack. The warm, humid environment reduces airway drying and irritation, leading to fewer asthma symptoms. Some exceptions would be chlorine sensitivity and certain physical allergies. If you have chlorine sensitivity or aquagenic urticaria, water aerobics is not the best choice. Aquatic classes provide good cardiovascular and pulmonary conditioning. Depth of the water can change the intensity of the workout and also change the workload, ranging from a lower-extremity to a whole-body workout. The water depth will also determine the stress placed on the joints with deeper water, chest or neck height, providing more buoyancy and less stress on the joints. The water temperature should be warm to avoid complications with cold urticaria and avoid airway cooling, which leads to airway irritation and asthma symptoms. Never join a class if no lifeguard is on duty. The same principles of exercise intensity, duration, and frequency apply to water aerobics and are discussed later. Some land classes may meet outside, so make sure to monitor the humidity, temperature, pollen counts, and air pollution before participating in an outdoor class. See chapter 7 for more information on exercise environment.

Aerobics classes, land or water based, should last between 30 and 60 minutes depending on the level of the class. The total class time should include an adequate warm-up and cool-down. Beginners should start out with 5 to 10 minutes of warm-up, continue with 15 to 20 minutes of low-intensity aerobic exercise, and end with a 5- to 10-minute cool-down. A more active, fit person may look for a class with a high-intensity, 35- to 40-minute aerobic session and similar warm-up and cool-down periods. Beginners should exercise only three sessions a week and advance to five sessions a week as aerobic capacity improves. Be careful of exercising too frequently; overuse injuries often occur. Any given aerobics session should not last more than 60 minutes. You may adjust the frequency and duration of your sessions according to your desired fitness goals, allowing for at least one or two days for rest and strength training.

The aerobics instructor is vital in determining your satisfaction and safety in your land or water aerobics class. Ask your instructor about his or her qualifications. Several fitness councils and governing bodies offer certification for strength and conditioning instructors. Find out whether your instructor is certified and by whom. An experienced instructor will understand how to adjust an activity to meet your specific needs. Notify the instructor of your asthma or EIA. Aquatic and land instructors should have basic CPR certification or a lifeguard should be on duty during your aquatic exercise session. Always have your rescue inhaler handy, and premedicate 10 to 15 minutes before you exercise. If you are experiencing asthma symptoms or your peak flow is not optimal, sit out and try again the next day at a lower intensity level. Know your limitations, and choose your class based on individual goals and level of fitness.

Stationary Cycling

Stationary cycling (sometimes known by the trademarked name Spinning) classes are really aerobics classes using a stationary bicycle. These classes emulate a road cycling session. If you have asthma, EIA, or allergies and the weather is either too dry or too cold and the pollen count or air quality is not favorable, stationary cycling classes are an ideal way to add cycling to your exercise program. Stationary cycling will improve your exercise tolerance and aerobic capacity just as outdoor cycling will. However, the controlled environment, including no road safety concerns, should allow you to cycle when outdoor conditions are suboptimal. Another advantage to stationary cycling is the ease at which you may monitor your heart rate to determine your level of exercise intensity.

Cycling classes usually last 40 minutes. Classes come in varying intensities, and the intensity of the class is determined by the percentage of target heart rate achieved by the participants. Lower-level classes will start out at 50 to 60 percent of target heart rate, and more intense classes may stress you to 60 to 80 percent. The 40-minute duration is based on the ACSM guideline of 20 to 30 minutes of aerobic exercise, 3 to 5 times a week (ACSM 2005). The session includes a 5- to 10-minute warm-up and cool-down and at least 20 minutes of endurance training. Your exercise intensity will vary with pedal resistance, pedal speed, handlebar position, and body position in the saddle. If you have never tried stationary cycling, you should start with a beginner class. Proper position on the bike is important. Your seat should be high enough that your leg is only slightly bent with your foot on the pedal. Your arms should rest comfortably on the handlebars and slightly flex at the elbow. Start with the handlebars in a higher position. As you improve you may lower the handlebars. Ask the instructor to evaluate your seat and handlebar position as well as your posture on the bike. Keeping your head, neck, and spine in good alignment will reduce discomfort and prevent injury.

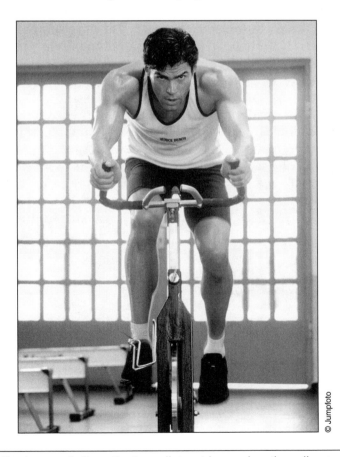

© Jumpfoto

Stationary cycling is a great alternative to cycling outdoors when the pollen count is high.

Cycling classes are very lively and full of energy, but stationary cycling is not a race. If you experience coughing, wheezing, chest discomfort, or breathlessness, reduce your pedal speed and return to a seated position. If you are still having these problems, stop and check your peak flow rate. You should always have your rescue inhaler handy. Notify the instructor that you will be cycling at a lower level of intensity at the next class. An experienced instructor should be aware of each class member's needs and limitations. The instructor may call your name and instruct you to slow down, sit down, or stop. Before starting a class, inform the instructor of your asthma or EIA and inquire about his or her qualifications. If you have any doubts about your fitness level and ability to participate in a cycling class, consult your physician.

Summary

Exploring alternative exercise classes will diversify your exercise routine and should improve your overall fitness. Many of these exercise classes are popular and will likely improve your aerobic capacity. These classes all differ in the area of conditioning and fitness that they stress. Adding one of these classes to a traditional exercise program can focus on improving one area of fitness. On the other hand, these classes can combine multiple fitness and conditioning aspects to provide a more holistic slant to a traditional exercise program. These classes should serve as adjuncts to traditional exercise programs, especially in the setting of asthma or EIA. Too little scientific evidence exists supporting these alternative classes to supplant traditional aerobic exercise as the best exercise form to improve asthma or EIA symptoms. You can be assured of the safety of these programs if you choose your class based on your current fitness level, follow appropriate medication regimens, and choose a qualified fitness instructor. I hope these guidelines will help you choose the appropriate alternative exercise class. Enjoy your new class, and continue your quest to stay fit.

EXPLORING ALTERNATIVE FORMS OF EXERCISE

☐ Remember that alternative exercise forms are just that—alternative. They are not intended to replace traditional aerobic exercise or strength training programs.

☐ Be aware that, while likely beneficial, some alternative exercise forms have only minimal scientific evidence of benefit to allergies, asthma, and EIA.

☐ Follow the same principles of warm-up, cool-down, duration, frequency, and intensity with alternative exercise programs as discussed for cardiovascular programs in chapter 3.

☐ Choose your classes and instructors carefully; do your homework.

☐ Always monitor your peak flow, follow your appropriate medication regimen, and notify the instructor of your condition.

☐ Enjoy yourself!

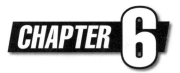

MANAGING ALLERGIES THROUGH TOLERANCE AND DESENSITIZATION

William Briner

In general, you can best manage allergic symptoms and maintain your exercise regimen by taking your medication before exercise sessions. However, allergy management methods exist that do not involve prescription or over-the-counter medicines, and they work for some people. These methods involve tolerance and the immune system. As tolerance occurs, the body's immune system essentially becomes used to an allergen, and that allergen becomes less likely to provoke symptoms. Desensitization is the medical application of tolerance through a physician's office. For instance, successful desensitization may allow a person who had previously reacted to the presence of cats with sneezing and watery eyes to be able to exercise without problems in a house where cats are kept.

Food allergies occur in about 1 to 2 percent of adults and up to 8 percent of children. These allergies in exercisers are discussed at the end of the chapter. An elimination diet may help to identify allergenic foods. This type of diet involves eliminating a given food from the diet and seeing whether allergic symptoms resolve. The safest management for food allergy is avoidance of foods known to cause allergic reactions. Severe anaphylactic reactions may necessitate a need for medical desensitization from food allergy as well. Exercise may worsen food allergy symptoms because increased peripheral blood flow as the muscles contract may result in more systemic exposure to the ingested antigen. Individuals with a known food allergy may therefore wish to avoid exercise for several hours after eating.

Implementing Tolerance

From a medical perspective, tolerance is the immune system phenomenon that occurs with progressively increasing exposures to an allergen over time. Initially a tiny amount of allergen (such as pollen) is used. Then over several weeks, the amount of allergen is increased. With repeated exposures, an amount of allergen that previously would have produced symptoms no longer does so. The body's immune system has become tolerant to that allergen. Desensitization is the medical application of tolerance. First, the precise allergen that produces symptoms, such as bee sting venom, is identified. Then a minimal dose of this substance is injected under sterile conditions beneath the skin. Each week the injection is repeated with gradually increasing doses of venom. After several weeks to months, a bee sting will no longer result in a severe reaction.

Avoidance

Any discussion of allergen exposure should start with avoidance. This is basically the commonsense idea that substances that are likely to produce allergic symptoms are best avoided if possible. For instance, someone who is allergic to cats should avoid exercising in a home where cats reside. If you know that you have a hay fever reaction to ragweed pollen, you should exercise indoors in the fall months. This method is obviously far easier for managing symptoms than a long course of multiple injections. Nonetheless, some people would rather not change their environment. For example, some people visit allergists for desensitization shots rather than removing pets from their homes. From a medical standpoint, this decision is difficult to defend. The safest and most straightforward principle to follow in allergy management is the principle of avoidance. Following this simple advice will help to decrease the need for expensive medication and the chance of life-threatening allergic reaction.

Tolerance and Exercise

You may use the principle of tolerance to gradually decrease allergic symptoms during exercise. In other words, if you have suffered respiratory allergic symptoms or asthma with exercise, you may be able to decrease these symptoms if you start slowly and very gradually increase your exercise duration and intensity.

This principle applies best to exercise-induced asthma (EIA). For instance, say a given runner experiences wheezing and coughing after running for 12 minutes at a 6-minute-per-mile pace. If she starts by running at a pace of 8 minutes a mile and runs only 10 minutes on her first day of training, then she can gradually speed up her pace and increase the time spent running with each training session. After 10 days or so, she will be able to train for 20 minutes at her desired pace without symptoms.

Athletes with EIA who do a moderate-intensity warm-up about a half hour before anticipated strenuous activity will be able to exercise longer and more strenuously without symptoms. Their airways probably become tolerant of the large volumes of relatively cool, dry air inspired during exercise. You can use this warm-up effect in practice and competition settings to decrease the likelihood and severity of EIA. A sample program to induce tolerance in EIA follows.

Sample Exercise Tolerance Program

Here is a sample program to induce exercise tolerance in a runner with EIA who wishes to compete in 10K races:

▸ In his best 10K race, he ran at a 7-minute-per-mile pace, but he was wheezing throughout the second half of the race.

▸ He must take two puffs of albuterol 15 minutes before *every* training session and competition.

If he ever notices wheezing during a run or cough afterward, he should return to the previous day's workout for 2 days and then try again to increase his activity.

Day 1: 4 miles at 8-minute-per-mile pace

Day 2: 5 miles at 8-minute-per-mile pace

Day 3: 6 miles at 8-minute-per-mile pace

Day 4: 7 miles at 8-minute-per-mile pace

Day 5: 5 miles at 7.5-minute-per-mile pace

Day 6: 6 miles at 8-minute-per-mile pace

Day 7: off

Day 8: 4 miles at 7-minute-per-mile pace

Day 9: 5 miles at 7-minute-per-mile pace

Day 10: 6 miles at 7-minute-per-mile pace

Day 11: 7 miles at 7.5-minute-per-mile pace

Day 12: 4 miles at 7.5-minute-per-mile pace

Day 13: off—easy 1-hour bike ride with friends

Day 14: Race day: warm-up: jog at a 10-minute-per-mile pace for 8 minutes, 30 minutes before race. Compete at 6.5-minute-per-mile pace.

You have many good reasons to stick to your exercise program. Both the cardiovascular and strength training effects are lost rather quickly when exercise behavior ceases. Whatever your allergic response is, and whatever allergen causes it, tolerance to exercise in the environment that provokes an allergic response is maintained only if the exercise behavior is maintained. If the runner in this example takes a 2-month break from exercise, he will almost certainly start wheezing again at 3 miles when he returns to running.

Choosing From Among Aerobic Options

You can use the principles of avoidance and tolerance when choosing a type (mode) of aerobic exercise that is less likely to cause symptoms. The correct type of cardiovascular activity is the one that you enjoy doing and that gives you satisfaction from completing your workout. As noted, it is almost always possible for people with allergies to participate in whatever sport desired if they pay attention to triggers for their symptoms and take their medication in a timely fashion. However, if minimizing allergic symptoms is a primary focus for you and the mode of exercise is less of a priority, some factors with respect to allergic conditions may guide your choice of activity.

EIA symptoms are more likely to occur with inhalation of cold, dry air. So running outside in temperatures below 40 degrees Fahrenheit would be a poor choice for someone with EIA. Swimming, a sport in which warm, moist air is inhaled, is a better option. Outdoor exercise may likewise be easier to tolerate for people with EIA if they take steps to prepare for

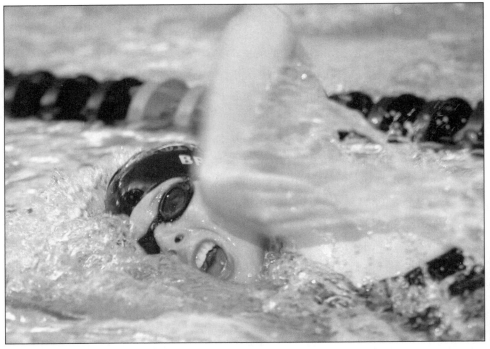

© 2006 Stacie Freudenberg

If cold air sets off your EIA symptoms, try swimming indoors—the air at the pool is usually warm and humid.

aerobic activity in the cold. Anything that helps to warm inhaled air will decrease the likelihood of an attack, so a mask or scarf that covers the mouth and nose should be helpful. A chief function of the nasal airway is warming and humidifying inhaled air, so nose breathing as much as possible during exercise will minimize EIA symptoms as well.

Some of the advice with respect to exercise options is just common sense. If you know that you are sensitive to indoor dust and molds, then outdoor activities are the choice for you. If sulfur dioxide from auto emissions is likely to touch off an asthma attack and you live in a large city, then indoor treadmill running may be a better aerobic activity. Some people may be able to exercise outdoors on certain days if they pay close attention to allergens such as air pollution and pollen levels on a day-to-day basis.

Considering Desensitization

The question of desensitization (or immunotherapy) shots is a difficult one for primary care physicians and allergists to address. Many of the people who think they may benefit from a desensitization program have not had a life-threatening allergic event. The shots don't work for everyone, and multiple shots are necessary for even a chance of effectiveness.

The decision to administer allergy shots is easier to make in people who have had severe systemic allergic reactions. For instance, a soccer player who has had anaphylaxis to a bee sting should have desensitization shots if he must continue playing outdoors. Anaphylaxis is the most extreme sort of hypersensitivity allergic reaction. The substances released into the bloodstream during this reaction (histamine, leukotrienes) cause the smooth muscle in the small blood vessels to relax. The vessels become much wider across (dilate), and blood pressure drops (vascular collapse). Anaphylaxis may cause a person to pass out or even die.

Angioedema is an acute allergic reaction that results in swelling of the hands, feet, face, lips, and throat. Swelling of the larynx may become so severe that the airway closes off and death may occur. People who have had one anaphylaxis or angioedema reaction have a 50 percent chance of experiencing such a systemic reaction the next time they are exposed to that allergen. If they cannot with certainty avoid exposure to the allergen they are hypersensitive to, they should strongly consider desensitization shots.

Some question may exist as to what constitutes a systemic reaction. For instance, a bee sting may result in impressive swelling of the entire forearm. Most physicians agree that a systemic reaction is one in which swelling in the arm includes the entire upper extremity and spreads across the midline of the body. In these cases, immunotherapy should be considered. Those who have had severe local reactions should be followed closely, because repeated exposures to the same allergen may result in a heightened immune response and more severe symptoms with repeated exposures. They should avoid exposure to known allergens as much as possible.

Other asthma and hay fever cases exist where immunotherapy injections may help someone to continue exercising. They may include people in whom medications (antihistamines and inhalers) do not work to control symptoms or those who have side effects from the medications. If these side effects are so severe that the person cannot take any effective medication, then desensitization may be a reasonable consideration.

In general, immunotherapy is effective in about 3 out of 4 people with hay fever and in about 9 out of 10 people with bee sting allergy. Typically weekly shots are necessary for many months. Shots are administered subcutaneously (under the skin). A physician must take special care to observe the patient closely for severe systemic reactions, especially with the initial series of injections. These reactions must be treated immediately if they occur. If the shots are effective, then less frequent doses may be administered. Sometimes occasional maintenance doses may be necessary over several years. Recently, immunotherapy using sublingual (under the tongue) application of allergens has been evaluated in medical studies. It may be that this method of desensitization will be useful in the future, without the need for injections. People with asthma that is not well controlled with prescription medicines and who are known to have allergic triggers for their asthma may also benefit from desensitization.

The choice to have an evaluation for desensitization shots in a physician's office can be a difficult one. Depending on the type of allergen and how the immunotherapy is studied, effectiveness may vary between 50 and 90 percent. Immunotherapy itself is not without risk. Severe reactions, including anaphylaxis, can occur as side effects of the treatment. Again, it probably does not make sense to be evaluated for the allergens that cause your symptoms unless you have severe allergic symptoms and you would be willing to undergo a series of desensitization shots lasting months to years if it were indicated. If you would object to having the multiple injections necessary to treat your allergic reaction, then you probably have no reason to undergo an extensive allergy evaluation. If you do elect to undergo such evaluation, a couple of options are available.

RAST   A radioallergosorbent test (RAST) is a blood test that identifies hypersensitivity to common antigens. These might include pollens or pet dander. The RAST is fairly accurate. Some physicians use it to initiate and monitor immunotherapy. It has the advantages of being rapid and necessitating only a single needle stick to draw blood.

Skin Testing   This involves placing a small amount of the suspected allergen on the skin, and then scratching the skin with a sterile needle, which injects a tiny amount of the allergen into the skin. Swelling and redness indicate a type I hypersensitivity reaction. Skin testing has the advantages of being more sensitive and specific for individual allergens. Response to therapy may also be easier and more accurately followed with skin testing.

Dealing With Food Allergy

Food allergy is a fairly common condition affecting as many as 2.7 million Americans. Some very rare instances exist when food sensitivity may be directly related to exercise and allergy. Exercise-induced anaphylaxis may be more likely to occur after ingestion of shellfish, wheat, or any food in some people diagnosed with this condition. Therefore, people known to have exercise-induced anaphylaxis should wait 4 hours after eating before they exercise.

Two types of adverse food reactions exist. Food intolerance probably accounts for the majority of adverse reactions and is most likely a reaction to food additives such as preservatives and dyes. True allergic reactions to food would be classified as food hypersensitivities. They are most common early in life, with a prevalence as high as 8 percent in children less than 3 years of age (Bock 1987). It seems that most people grow out of their food allergies, because their prevalence in adulthood is probably closer to 1 percent. Peanut allergy, in particular, seems to be increasing in America in recent years.

Food Allergens

Sensitization to food allergens may occur after food is ingested or after exposure to inhaled antigens. Fortunately, the walls of the stomach and intestine have a lining of mucus. This mucosal barrier helps to keep antigenic proteins from being absorbed through the gut and helps to prevent systemic allergic reactions to ingested food. Cow's milk is usually the first foreign protein introduced into an infant's diet.

Cow's milk allergy is a fairly common form of childhood food allergy. Humans can form antibodies to at least 20 proteins in cow's milk. Chicken eggs cause the greatest number of allergic reactions in children. Peanuts are the most common food allergy beyond 4 years of age. Soybeans may also precipitate allergic reactions in children and adults.

Tree nuts (walnuts, cashews, almonds, pecans, and pistachios) may also cause allergic reactions. Shellfish, including the mollusks (snails, mussels, scallops, and oysters) as well as the crustaceans (lobsters, crabs, and shrimp) can induce food allergy. Wheat and other grains contain several proteins that may be antigenic. Prolifin is a protein that has been identified in several fruits and vegetables as an allergenic protein.

Symptoms of Food Hypersensitivity

The oral allergy syndrome is a common manifestation of food allergy, particularly for plant proteins. It is common among adults with respiratory allergy to pollen. The usual symptoms are tingling and itchiness (pruritus) of the mouth, throat, lips, and tongue. Less commonly, swelling (angioedema) may occur. Symptoms usually last only a few minutes and then resolve spontaneously. Treatment is rarely necessary.

Gastrointestinal anaphylaxis is a more severe form of food allergy in which nausea, vomiting, abdominal pain, and diarrhea occur within minutes to hours after ingesting the antigenic food. Symptoms usually subside within 24 hours. Fever is usually not seen. This condition seems to occur more commonly in children with atopic dermatitis (eczema). Hives may also rarely occur as a result of food allergy.

Evaluation and Treatment of Food Allergy

The most effective way to figure out what food is causing the allergic symptoms is usually an elimination diet. History of symptoms following exposure to certain foods known to be allergenic may help suggest what food to eliminate. If it is not readily apparent, then keeping a diary of foods eaten and symptoms noted over one to several weeks may be helpful. Then, the potentially offending food is eliminated from the diet for 2 weeks. If no symptoms occur, an oral challenge of a tiny amount of that food may be ingested. If less severe symptoms occur, then the diagnosis is fairly certain. Skin-prick testing and RAST may be helpful in some situations as well.

As is the case for many types of allergy, the safest and easiest way to deal with food allergy is avoidance. A person with known severe food allergy should avoid exercise for 3 to 4 hours after eating to possibly prevent a more severe systemic reaction. After an offending food has been identified, the best advice is simply not to ever ingest that food again. Obviously, this reaction becomes more of a priority with a history of more severe allergic reactions such as angioedema or anaphylaxis. In rare situations, an oral or subcutaneous injection desensitization program to a food allergen can be successfully undertaken.

Summary

Exercisers can use the immune system phenomena of tolerance and desensitization to control their allergies, sometimes without the need for medication. Tolerance occurs with successive exposures to an allergen over time, resulting in a lesser degree of symptoms with each exposure. Tolerance may be particularly useful in controlling EIA. The warm-up effect (wherein strenuous exercise is less likely to elicit an EIA attack after a less intense warm-up) is a manifestation of tolerance. Desensitization is the medical application of tolerance under a physician's guidance. This procedure is clearly indicated for exercisers who have had life-threatening allergic reactions to fairly common allergen exposures. A baseball player with severe bee sting allergy might be an example. Larger and larger doses of antigen are given over time, and, if desensitization is effective, the person will no longer react to that antigen after a series of shots. While these techniques are useful, the safest and easiest allergy management technique remains avoidance. If known provocative allergens or allergy provoking situations can possibly be avoided, symptoms can be prevented.

Food allergy is fairly common in both adults and children. Cow's milk, peanuts, and shellfish are some of the foods likely to cause symptoms. Symptoms may include the oral allergy syndrome, with itching and tingling noted in the mouth, lips, and throat. Food allergy may also manifest as stomach pain, vomiting, and diarrhea. Sometimes it is difficult to identify the offending food. Eliminating the food item that might possibly be causing symptoms and observing what happens may be useful (elimination diet). Avoidance of known allergy-causing foods is the best therapeutic option.

ACTION PLAN:
MANAGING ALLERGIES THROUGH TOLERANCE AND DESENSITIZATION

- ☐ Warm up prior to intense exercise if you have exercise-induced asthma. It may decrease your chance of symptoms.
- ☐ If you have had a life-threatening allergic reaction to an insect sting, see a physician for desensitization to insect sting venom.
- ☐ Avoid known allergens if possible.
- ☐ Try to identify the cause of food allergy symptoms by eliminating the suspected food and observing to see whether symptoms subside.
- ☐ Avoid foods known to cause allergic symptoms.

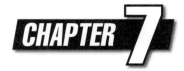

CHAPTER 7

CREATING AN ALLERGEN-FREE ENVIRONMENT

Matthew J. Brandon

An estimated 30 percent of the United States population has some type of allergic condition. The cost to society is far greater than you may think when you factor in the cost of medication, absenteeism, emergency room visits, physician appointments, and comorbid conditions worsened by allergic conditions. It is a well-established theory and practice that avoiding allergens by modifying the home environment will prevent the frequency and severity of allergic conditions. This practice is routinely stressed in the daily care of people with asthma, especially the pediatric population. The same may be said for avoiding outdoor allergens. Unfortunately, people often overlook the importance of the exercise environment when starting or modifying an exercise program. All too often people select an exercise location based on factors that have no effect on the body's physiologic response to exercise. Naturally, psychosocial elements, convenience, cost, equipment, and aesthetics are major factors in choosing an exercise location. If you have allergic rhinitis, physical allergies, exercise-induced asthma (EIA), or asthma, choosing an exercise location based on the aforementioned factors is not wise. Those elements are important too, but being aware of the effect of allergens, air pollutants, and climate on exercise will help ensure a safe and enjoyable exercise experience.

The dark, dank, drafty free-weight room may be a rugged and hip place to lift weights, but this location is likely teeming with indoor allergens waiting to expose themselves to your upper airway, skin, mucous membranes, and eyes. The same may be said for your home gym, except you can probably add pet allergens and dust mites to the allergen list. You're probably saying to yourself, *I'll just exercise outside.* Not so fast. You really need to be careful with outdoor exercise; each season brings on new allergens, not to mention changing temperatures, humidity, and air pollution. However, don't be scared. By now you understand all the benefits of exercise for allergic conditions and are convinced of the safety of exercising with allergic conditions. You should use the information in this chapter to further improve your current exercise environment or choose an appropriate environment to begin exercise. Previous chapters have emphasized the safety, benefits, and treatment of asthma, EIA, allergic rhinitis, and physical allergies as they relate to exercise. Preventing environmental allergy is just as important. A close friend of mine was experiencing congestion, headache, and cough while running on his treadmill. Simply moving the treadmill from the basement and changing his home's humidity level greatly improved his symptoms. I personally found triathlon training in the spring very difficult because of allergic rhinitis. Now, I always watch the pollen and air quality indexes and choose to swim on days when the numbers are suboptimal. How do *you* prevent allergies? The answer is simple: Avoid the allergens and climatic factors that exacerbate your allergic conditions.

In the past two decades several new and better treatments for allergic conditions have become available. Despite improved understanding and treatment of allergy, prevalence of allergic disease has reached epidemic proportions. Exposure to indoor and outdoor environmental allergens is probably a contributor. Athletes and other active people pose a unique problem with managing allergic conditions. First, athletes are often exposed to outdoor elements and allergens during multiple seasons. To that end, physical activity increases ventilation rate, allowing even more exposure to the elements and allergens. As mentioned in previous chapters, allergic conditions can reduce performance in multiple ways and sometimes can result in more serious or even fatal conditions. Many studies, including studies of Olympic athletes, have shown a high prevalence of allergic disease in athletes. You may be in the same situation. Your personal physician is always the best source of information and guidance for managing your allergies, but you certainly can take steps to improve your indoor environment and monitor the outdoor environment to avoid days with suboptimal air quality, pollen counts, mold spore counts, or other weather conditions.

Common Airborne Allergens

▸ Tree pollen

▸ Grass pollen

▸ Weed pollen

▸ Wet mold spores

▸ Dry mold spores

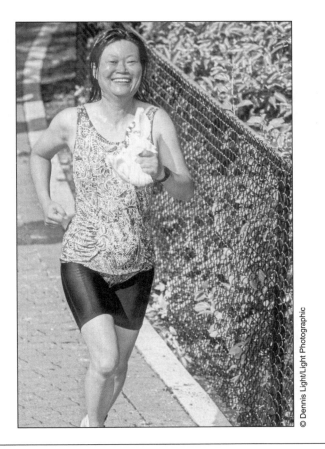

Exercising outdoors can help you get away from the mold and dust of indoor exercise environments, as long as the air quality is good and the pollen counts are low.

As discussed in previous chapters, you can choose to exercise in two basic environments: indoor and outdoor. As a whole, our society spends a great deal of time indoors. The majority of indoor climates are affected by central air conditioning, central heating, carpet, insulation, and low ventilation. The net effects of decreased ventilation are increased moisture, humidity, and molds. Certainly, the moisture fluctuates with heating and air conditioning, but overall our homes are less ventilated and more moist than previously. The number of homes with indoor pets has increased over the years. Our ever-increasing standard of living has brought pets indoors and pet allergens with them. Dogs, cats, birds, and other pets will certainly increase your home's allergen count exponentially. Also because we are spending more time indoors, we are exposed to the ubiquitous dust mite and cockroach allergens. Yes, as clean as your house may be, you probably still have dust mites and cockroach allergens. The allergens mentioned here are the usual suspects for allergic rhinitis, EIA, and asthma. Several mechanisms have been proposed and studied to limit or rid the home or

Common Air Pollutants

▸ Ozone

▸ Tobacco smoke

▸ Fine particulate matter

▸ Diesel exhaust particles

▸ Nitrogen dioxide

▸ Sulfur dioxide

indoor environment of dust mite allergens, cockroach allergens, pet allergens, and mold spores. Physical allergies from temperature, water, and sunlight may also affect you during exercise.

The outdoor environment has also evolved as our society has evolved. Industrialization, the internal-combustion engine, aerosols, air travel, and other technological advances have all influenced our air quality. The sidebar on this page details multiple air pollutants. These pollutants can increase acute response to allergens, resulting in higher sensitivity to outdoor allergens. Internal-combustion engines create diesel particle pollutants. Avoiding construction sites and busy roads and steering clear of gas-powered lawn mowers will improve your exercise environment. Organic particulate matter includes tree pollens, grass pollens, and weed pollens. In some climates pollens may be associated with certain seasons. Weather, such as thunderstorms or rain showers, may affect the prevalence of pollen on any given day. Fungal spores are also ubiquitous in the outdoor environment except for the extremely cold or arctic environments. Spores generally live in fields or wooded areas and tend to thrive in damp environments. Spores are present throughout most of the year with peaks during different seasons. As if you didn't have enough to think about, the great outdoors brings nonallergic variables, including wind, air temperature, sunlight, and humidity. These variables can affect allergic conditions by changing the moisture and temperature of the skin, mucous membranes, and airway, resulting in exaggerated response to allergens. In addition, changes in these variables can increase or decrease the concentration of pollen and mold spores in the air. Although outdoor climate can be quite constant, geographically speaking, even small changes or microclimates can vary the allergen and spore counts significantly (see table 7.1). Any sudden change in climate conditions may cause early and late changes in the allergen counts. For instance, the mold count may increase the first day or so of a windy season (early change), but the overall mold count may not significantly rise when looking at the entire windy season (late change). The same may be said of rainy seasons. The pollen and mold counts may not be affected the first few days of the rainy season (early change), but when considering the entire rainy season length, the counts generally will rise (late change). A thunderstorm in an arid region or a cool, damp valley near a stream in the same arid region will certainly produce allergen counts that differ greatly from the region norms. Exercise outdoors during low-allergen days or seasons and in climates traditionally low in allergen count will improve your performance and help you stick to your exercise program.

Table 7.1   Climatic Effects on Allergens

Variable	Pollen		Mold	
	Early change	Late change	Early change	Late change
Humidity ↑	Lower	Unknown	Higher	Higher
Temperature ↑	Higher	Higher	Higher	Higher
Rain ↑	Equivocal	Higher	Equivocal	Higher
Wind ↑	Higher	Higher	Higher	Equivocal

Reprinted from *Immunology and Allergy Clinics of North America,* Vol. 23, R.W. Weber, "Meteorologic variables in aerobiology," pp. 411-422, Copyright 2003, with permission from Elsevier.

Indoor Environment

The home has evolved into more than a place to rest your head. In fact, most of our homes are offices, meeting places, day care centers, and personal exercise gyms. Fortunately you have some control over your home environment. You should optimize your home exercise environment so that you can enjoy your step aerobics video, treadmill, recumbent bicycle, or other exercise equipment. You may be thinking that exercising at home should be no problem because you haven't experienced significant wheezing, coughing, or congestion at home. It seems logical, but how often do you breathe deeply 20 to 30 times a minute during a regular day at home? Probably not very often. This is precisely why home exercise will increase your exposure to the allergens listed in table 7.2. The advantage to exercising at home, in addition to cost and convenience, is the ability to manipulate your environment to reduce your allergen exposure.

You can reduce your exposure to indoor allergens by following some simple guidelines. Your indoor exercise space should not be in the basement or the garage. The basement tends to be moist and harbors mold and mold

Table 7.2   Common Allergens in Skin Testing

Indoor allergens	Outdoor allergens
Dust mite *(D. farinae)*	Bermuda grass
Dust mite *(D. pteronyssinus)*	Sweet vernal grass
Cat pelt	Rye grass
Cat hair	Timothy grass
	Ragweed
	Red top grass

spores. The garage tends to be loaded with air pollutants from oil, gasoline, and other noxious fumes. Choosing an area at ground level is ideal. Exercising in a converted attic or upper level can be very hot or cold depending on the season or time of day. Try to keep your pets out of the exercise room. Carpet, pillows, stuffed animals, and stuffed furniture harbor dust mites and pet allergens and should not be in your exercise room. Also, limit the number of plants in your home and exercise room to reduce the amount of mold and fungus. Your exercise room should be well ventilated, provided your home ventilation system has an adequate air filtration system and no moisture buildup. Ventilation to the outdoor environment can expose you to outdoor allergens, including pollen, pollutants, and mold spores. If your home is equipped with the technology, one of the best features of exercising at home is the ability to adjust air humidity and temperature. Keeping the humidity level between 30 and 50 percent should help reduce some of the perennial indoor allergens. Avoid extremes of temperature and humidity; an exceedingly dry or cold indoor environment will increase mucous membrane and airway sensitivity to allergens. Another advantage of exercising in your home is the absence of wind. Wind dries the mucous membranes and airway, increasing the sensitivity to allergens. Tobacco smoke is both an allergen and an airway irritant. Do not allow anyone to smoke in your home, and especially ban smoking in your exercise room. If you currently smoke, I recommend consulting your personal physician for smoking cessation options. You can prevent physical allergy symptoms by choosing an exercise location with limited exposure to the offending allergen. For example, placing your treadmill in front of a big bay window may not be a good idea if you have solar urticaria.

Allergy Testing

You can take several steps to reduce allergens in your home to improve or prevent allergic conditions when exercising. It is always wise to attempt to reduce the perennial allergens listed previously in table 7.2. To that end, you should consider allergy testing to determine your specific sensitivities so that you can remove these allergens from your home. If you have persistent allergic symptoms after taking steps to avoid allergen exposure and you are adhering to your medication regimen, allergy testing is probably a good idea. The science behind allergy testing is discussed in chapter 6. Allergen skin testing is usually performed for airborne allergens in individuals with recalcitrant allergic rhinitis or asthma but may also be important in food, insect sting, and medication allergy. Skin testing may consist of as many as 40 allergens; the most common of these allergens are listed in table 7.2. As mentioned in chapter 6, serum IgE (an immune system protein partially responsible for allergen sensitivity) levels can be identified for specific allergens by performing RAST testing on blood samples. This method of testing may be useful if skin testing is not an option because of severe skin conditions, ongoing medical treatment, or the possibility of life-threatening anaphylaxis. Allergy testing will assist you in identifying both indoor and outdoor allergens that may affect your exercise performance.

Dust Mites

Dust mites are the most common indoor allergen and have been the topic of a vast array of scientific study. Dust mite concentration and exposure have correlated with the prevalence and severity of asthma and allergic rhinitis. House dust mites and their excrement are found in bed sheets, carpets, stuffed furniture, mattresses, pillows, stuffed animals, and other textiles commonly found around your home. Dust mites thrive in damp conditions. Keeping the humidity level between 40 and 50 percent will reduce dust mite concentration. Choosing to exercise in a well-ventilated, low-humidity room will reduce your exposure while exercising.

The most effective method of reducing your exposure to dust mites is to pick up your belongings and move to the mountains. An altitude above 5,000 feet and low humidity make mountain living a great choice for reducing exposure to dust mite allergens. Although effective, moving to a high altitude is obviously impractical for most of us. To reduce dust mites, you should use impenetrable covers for mattresses, pillows, and comforters. These covers do not allow the mites access to food sources, and they perish. Avoid exercising in your bedroom. Dust mites accumulate more on rough, carpeted surfaces than on smooth floors. Removing carpet from your home will help reduce dust mite exposure. Definitely remove any carpet placed over concrete because the moisture level is higher and more favorable for dust mite accumulation. I recommend exercising in a noncarpeted room. Vacuuming and dusting once or twice a week will reduce dust mite accumulation. However, vacuuming and dusting can increase air concentration of dust mites for about 30 minutes. Use a filter mask or vacuum HEPA filter to decrease allergen exposure. Wait at least 30 minutes to exercise after vacuuming or dusting.

Washing bedroom linens weekly helps reduce dust mite allergen levels. You must wash linens at 130 degrees Fahrenheit or higher to kill dust mites. Exposing dust mites to air temperatures of 140 degrees Fahrenheit for several hours in a commercial dryer will reliably kill them. Chlorine bleach also will reduce dust mite allergen levels. Several chemical powders or sprays can be applied to furniture, carpet, or linens to reduce and kill dust mites. These methods are not uniform and have not conclusively demonstrated effectiveness. Reducing airborne dust mites is of particular interest to people who are sensitive and want to exercise. HEPA filters have been shown to reduce airborne dust mite allergen load. Also, commercially available dusting solutions may be used to reduce dust mite allergens in accumulated household dust. You can see why hopping on your treadmill in the damp, carpeted, poorly ventilated, recently vacuumed basement is probably not the best idea.

Pets

As stated previously, we are spending an increasing amount of our lives indoors. Our pets are too, and likely sitting right next to us. Dogs and cats have been linked to allergic rhinitis and asthma. I refer to dogs and cats throughout this section, but other pets with hair certainly carry similar risk. Clearly pets carry a large allergen load, and cats tend to be particularly allergen sensitizing. Pet allergens are usually found on smooth floors, carpets, furniture, and linens. Although considerably less than homes with pets, homes with no pets may have some amount of pet allergens from community pets. I have friends and family who see their pets as part of the family and could not bear the thought of removing them from the house. I still cannot convince one of my family members with asthma to remove the dogs from the home, although it is the simplest solution to reducing pet allergen exposure.

Short of giving Fido or Kitty the boot, you can reduce pet allergens by keeping your pets out of the bedroom and out of the designated exercise room. Follow the same vacuuming and dusting rules applied to dust mites. HEPA vacuum filters and HEPA air filters will also help reduce pet allergens, especially airborne pet allergens. HEPA filters are not an alternative to other allergen reduction measures, but they should be used as an adjunct method. Washing your pets and regularly grooming them can reduce allergen levels. Also, female cats produce less allergen load than their male counterparts. You may want to consider that fact before buying a new cat. If you follow these guidelines, you should be able to considerably reduce your pet allergen load. It is always a good idea to have allergy testing done to determine whether you are sensitive to your pet allergens.

Mold Spores

Mold spores are components of fungus reproduction. Mold spores have been associated with asthma and allergic rhinitis. The mold spores come in contact with skin, mucous membranes, and your airway when they become airborne. A majority of people with asthma are sensitive to mold spores. Reducing exposure to mold spores can prevent asthma and reduce asthma exacerbations.

How can you prevent mold growth in your house? Mold spore counts are much higher in the outdoor environment, and indoor mold spores likely come from the outdoor environment. Controlling humidity and moisture in your home will help reduce mold spores from accumulating. Keeping your home at less than 50 percent humidity should significantly reduce mold accumulation. Common areas for mold growth are the kitchen, basement, bathroom, and crawl space. During high outdoor mold spore counts keep windows and doors shut to reduce intrusion of mold spores from the outside. Increasing ventilation to the bathroom, kitchen, and basement can reduce moisture and humidity. Inspecting your home's foundation for cracks and subsequently repairing the cracks will reduce moisture and outdoor mold spore intrusion in your basement. Remove all carpets from concrete slabs. Remove household plants to reduce mold growth. Use chlorine bleach to clean mold-prone surfaces and help reduce mold growth. Other commercially available fungicides may work as well as bleach. Changing your furnace filter on a regular basis and having your furnace and duct work inspected for mold are also beneficial. Just remember, exercising in a poorly ventilated, damp, carpeted basement will certainly expose you to airborne mold. Allergen skin testing or serum IgE RAST testing can help you determine your sensitivity to specific mold species.

Cockroach Allergens

Cockroaches have been around since the dinosaurs and will likely continue to thrive. This news is not good for people with asthma and allergies because cockroaches are another perennial indoor allergen. Cockroach allergens exist in any household. The usual sites for cockroach allergen accumulation are the kitchen and kitchen cupboards, but you'll probably find cockroach allergens in all areas of the house. Reducing cockroach allergen load is difficult. Pesticide application followed by regular cleaning can reduce the allergen load for months, but eventually the populations will return. Storing food and water sources in sealed containers may help. Avoid accumulation of boxes and papers in kitchen cupboards and drawers. Cockroach allergen loads tend to be higher in lower socioeconomic homes and urban areas. Concrete construction is associated with higher cockroach allergen loads.

Reducing the allergen load in your home can improve your home exercise experience. You should strive for reduction of allergen levels and not total elimination, which is very difficult to achieve. If you choose to exercise indoors at a gym, evaluate the gym for the signs of favorable or unfavorable environmental conditions for exercise. Employing an organized approach to identifying your allergen sensitivity and reducing or preventing elevated home allergen levels will help ensure a safe and enjoyable home exercise experience (see table 7.3 for a summary of strategies).

Outdoor Environment

The outdoor environment is an inviting, exciting, and enjoyable place to exercise. The changing seasons, beautiful foliage, and other ever-changing climatic elements make the outdoors a great place to exercise, but these same elements may worsen allergic conditions. Elements such as wind, temperature, and humidity extremes can worsen allergic respiratory conditions as well. Throw in some air pollutants, and you may have a recipe for congestion, wheezing, coughing, rashes, or shortness of breath. The major players in outdoor allergens are grass pollen, tree pollen, plant pollen, and mold spores. Complicating the situation are air pollutants such as ozone, nitrogen dioxide, sulfur dioxide, particulate matter, and diesel exhaust particles that can aggravate allergic conditions. The best

Table 7.3   Indoor Environmental Modifications

	Dust mites	Pets	Mold spores	Cockroaches
Preventive steps	Use impervious mattress, pillow, blanket covers. Wash bedding in hot water weekly. Bleach bedding. Dry clean or tumble dry at high heat. Remove carpet. Increase home ventilation. Use HEPA air and vacuum filter. Use commercial dusting and cleaning solutions. Reduce humidity and temperature in home.	Remove pets from home. Remove pets from bedroom. Groom pets regularly. Remove carpet. Use HEPA air and vacuum filter. Use commercial dusting solutions. Choose female over male cats. Regularly dust and wipe smooth surfaces.	Close windows and doors during high-mold-count days. Bleach any moldy surfaces. Remove carpets and wash bathroom and kitchen rugs. Keep humidity level low. Remove indoor plants. Fix sources of standing water or moisture.	Use pesticides. Perform regular house cleaning. Tightly seal food sources before nighttime. Eliminate moisture in cupboards and kitchen. Remove cardboard boxes and paper bags.

way to minimize your exposure to outdoor allergens is to avoid exercising outside. If avoiding the outdoors is not feasible, you can adjust your exercise schedule based on time of day, your geographic location, pollen counts, air quality index, humidity levels, and temperature. Monitoring weather conditions for locations of specific events can help you pick the right event in a location favorable for your allergies. Your performance will probably be better and you'll be much happier picking an event in a low-allergen location. Following are some specifics on how to minimize exposure to allergens and pollutants.

Pollen

Many variables affect the amount of pollen in the air at any given time. The main variables affecting pollen release are season, humidity, rainfall, temperature, and wind speed. Pollen counts are generally higher in the late spring, summer, and early fall seasons. Precipitation has different effects on tree and grass pollen. Heavy thunderstorms with large raindrops may "scrub" the air of larger pollen grains while at the same time causing mechanical disturbance and release of pollen particles. Raindrops tend to scrub the large, nonbreathable pollen grains and may increase smaller, breathable pollen grains, creating a greater effect on asthma exacerbations over allergic rhinitis. The effect of thunderstorms seems to be related to mechanical release of pollen by wind and rain, settling of grass pollen from raindrops, and resuspension of pollen grains by higher wind velocities. Cumulative rainfall opposes the scrubbing effect by encouraging growth of grasses, weeds, and trees. Avoiding outdoor exercise during the days following cumulative rainfall may be wise. Thunderstorms are a unique situation that combines several weather elements to increase pollen counts. Generally lower humidity results in lower pollen counts as evidenced by the low pollen counts in arid climates. You still need to be conscious of the effect of airway drying when exercising in very low humidity and weigh the benefit of low pollen counts to the risk of dry air. Lower temperatures, especially temperatures producing frost, reduce grass and tree pollen counts significantly. The same risk–benefit formula should be applied to air temperature, especially if you have asthma. Conversely, cumulative high temperatures are signals for pollination, and higher pollen counts follow. These patterns are not true for all plants and trees; some are early or late pollinating species. Moderate to high wind speeds can increase airborne pollen counts, especially smaller grain tree pollens. Wind does not have as much of an effect on grass pollens. The double effect of airway drying and pollen exposure makes high winds problematic for active people with asthma.

Mold Spores

Exposure to mold spores is also a major concern if you have allergic conditions and exercise outdoors. Mold spores can be classified as dry or wet spores. Dry spores tend to be prevalent in more arid, windy, and warmer climates. Wet spores tend to be prevalent in damp areas and after cumulative rainfall. Allergy testing can help you determine your specific mold sensitivity. You may want to avoid exercising in dry, windy climates if you are sensitive to dry spores. Naturally, running or biking in a wooded coastal area may expose you to higher wet spore counts. Wet spores peak in the morning and dry spores peak in the afternoon, so adjust your exercise schedule according to your sensitivities. Mold counts tend to be higher in areas of dense foliage. Avoiding trail running or biking, for example, may reduce your exposure to mold. You're probably thinking, That's great, but running on the road has risks of traffic and higher air pollution. As with any recommendation, you need to look at all the factors in play and make adjustments by weighing risks and benefits.

Overall, it is a good idea to avoid exercise on days with high winds, higher temperatures, and especially days after cumulative rainfall and thunderstorms. Some of the most helpful information can be found in your local weather forecast. Pollen counts are often reported daily during spring, summer, and early fall. The NAB (National Allergy Bureau) scale, shown in table 7.4, will help you determine the pollen and mold counts for a specific day and location. I do not recommend exercising outdoors on days of high or very high pollen and mold counts. If you do choose to exercise outdoors, consider a filter mask and always take your medication. Allergy testing can help determine your specific allergen sensitization. This information can help you determine which time of year is least favorable for outdoor exercise. The American Academy of Allergy, Asthma, and Immunology Web site (www.aaaai.org) is an excellent source for information regarding outdoor and indoor allergens.

Table 7.4 Pollen and Mold Spore Counts

Mold spore		Grass pollen		Tree pollen		Weed pollen	
Count	Risk	Count	Risk	Count	Risk	Count	Risk
0	Absent	0	Absent	0	Absent	0	Absent
1-6,499	Low	1-4	Low	1-14	Low	1-9	Low
6,500-12,999	Moderate	5-19	Moderate	15-89	Moderate	10-49	Moderate
13,000-49,999	High	20-199	High	90-1,499	High	50-499	High
>50,000	Very high	>200	Very high	>1,500	Very high	>500	Very high

© American Academy of Allergy, Asthma & Immunology. All Rights Reserved.
Available: http://www.aaaai.org/nab/index.cfm?p=reading_charts [October 2005].

Air Pollutants

Air pollutants have been shown to worsen allergic rhinitis and asthma. The major air pollutants are as follows: ozone, tobacco smoke, fine particulate matter, and diesel exhaust particles. Smog is a product of photochemical reactions between ultraviolet radiation and vehicle exhaust emissions. Ozone is the most prevalent smog component. Ozone is ubiquitous but more prevalent in urban areas, around highways, and near industrial areas. Nitrogen dioxide and sulfur dioxide are also components of smog. These pollutants will reduce your airway's natural defense mechanisms with each breath. Ultraviolet light is required to produce smog. This requirement is precisely why these air pollutants are more prevalent on warm, summer days and in warmer climates. Diesel particulate matter is also a major cause of airway irritation and worsens allergic conditions. This pollutant also is more prevalent in urban areas and definitely in higher concentrations near roadways. Avoiding exercise in close proximity to gas-powered equipment will reduce the pollutants in your exercise environment. The United States Environmental Protection Agency produces an air quality index (AQI) that will help you determine air pollution levels on certain days (table 7.5). Avoiding outdoor exercise on days determined to be unhealthy is a wise choice.

Table 7.5 Air Quality Index

AQI index	Quality	Color scale
0-50	Good	Green
51-100	Moderate	Yellow
101-150	Unhealthy for sensitive groups	Orange
151-200	Unhealthy	Red
201-300	Very unhealthy	Purple
301-500	Hazardous	Maroon

Adapted from the U.S. Environmental Protection Agency, 2005. www.epa.gov.

Summary

Allergic rhinitis, EIA, and asthma are very common in active people. Athletic performance and physical activity may be adversely affected by uncontrolled allergic conditions. It is well established that avoiding allergens should be part of any treatment regimen for allergic conditions. Taking the appropriate steps to reduce your exposure to indoor and outdoor allergens will only serve to improve your physical performance and enhance your exercise experience. Reducing allergen exposure in your home is certainly under your control. Use the strategies detailed in this chapter to reduce your allergen exposure at home. Get comfortable using the pollen counts, mold spore counts, and air quality index to help modify your outdoor exercise schedule. Understanding allergen interaction with temperature, humidity, rainfall, wind, and air quality will be of great benefit to you in avoiding outdoor exercise during unfavorable conditions. Determining your specific allergen sensitivities can greatly improve your chances of avoiding specific allergens. To that end, you should still attempt to reduce your exposure to all perennial and seasonal allergens. Remember, your personal physician is an excellent source for information on how to avoid and prevent allergen exposure so that you can maintain your active lifestyle.

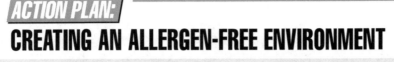

CREATING AN ALLERGEN-FREE ENVIRONMENT

- ☐ Remember that allergen avoidance is a key part of treating allergic conditions.
- ☐ Choose an appropriate indoor exercise space.
- ☐ Remove pets, carpet, and pillows from your exercise space.
- ☐ Use HEPA filters, but be aware that they are only adjuncts to more practical allergen removal recommendations.
- ☐ Monitor the pollen counts, mold counts, and air quality index to help you determine when outdoor exercise is more favorable.
- ☐ Consider allergen testing to help guide you in removing or avoiding a specific allergen.

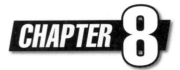

STAYING ON TRACK TO REDUCE SYMPTOMS

Jeffrey M. Mjaanes

Although planning and starting a new workout routine are challenging, most exercisers find sticking with the program is the hardest part. The excitement of starting a new adventure motivates people to begin working out. However, even advanced exercisers have difficulty maintaining their routine at times. Although you know and may even witness the benefits of exercise and staying fit, the motivation that helped you develop your routine sometimes wanes and you need a fresh wave of enthusiasm. As with most projects in life, staying on track can be difficult. Sometimes unavoidable and unexpected situations, such as illness or family emergencies, cause you to miss training days. Other times obstacles such as travel or busy schedules may interfere with your planned workouts. The key to sticking to your routine is not to try to work out through these hard times but to adapt to them, move on, and start your program again as soon as you are able.

Bouncing back after a break from working out is a common situation that may lead some people to give up their workouts all together. This situation is especially unfortunate in strength training because if you do not work out on a regular basis to at least maintain muscle tone, you will lose strength at a rate of 3 percent a week. Developing some tools to keep you motivated through the challenging times can help you maintain your gains and easily get right back into the game again. This chapter gives you some ideas on how to adapt your workout, roll with the punches as they say, and get back into your routine as soon as possible.

Avoiding Potential Pitfalls

You can address many challenges that interfere with your workout before you even start your program. Ask yourself a few simple questions. When will I work out? How often? Where will I train? Will the location be accessible? Will I need a workout partner, or can I motivate myself to work out alone?

Today we lead busy, fast-paced lives. Finding time to work out in our hectic daily schedules can be a challenge. It is best to plan a workout schedule ahead of time, choosing how many days a week you will train based on your goals. Decide how much time you will dedicate to each workout session and what time you will begin your workout. Leave a day each week as a catch-up day. If something comes up on your planned workout day, you can shift your training sessions by one and still be on target for the next week's workouts. Having a set schedule with some built-in flexibility time will help keep your training on track.

Finding an accessible exercise facility is also important. Choose a facility that is easy to get to from your home or work or both. If you drive to the gym, check whether parking is easily accessible and free or at least discounted. If you take public transportation to the gym, check the schedules for the times you will be going. Convenient hours are important. Many chain health clubs in larger cities now stay open late or even 24 hours. If the gym is far away or you have to drive around looking for parking and then walk a long distance, you might think it is easier to just stay home. To overcome these barriers, you must choose a fitness facility that is accessible in terms of location, parking, and hours.

Another helpful idea is to find a workout partner or friend who can reinforce your determination to train. Having someone who can work out with you will motivate you to keep going when the going gets tough. Many people find that making a commitment to a friend to meet at the gym at a certain time makes them less likely to skip a workout. In addition, that friend will help push them to complete each repetition and achieve gains they would not be able to do on their own. During exercises, a training partner can spot you to ensure you maintain proper form and can safely complete each repetition. Nevertheless, some people prefer to train by themselves. Many individuals enjoy the solitude of working out alone, choosing to focus their energy on their routine and not on socializing. Training alone also permits more flexibility in the scheduling of your workout since you are not dependent on anyone else's time. As a logical first step, you may also choose to try both options and then decide if working out alone or with a partner best suits your personality and training goals.

Planning Ahead for Allergies and Asthma

While you can never predict with absolute certainty when you are going to have an allergy flare-up or an asthma attack, you usually realize what triggers your exacerbations. Certain outdoor allergens, such as pollen or grasses; and indoor allergens, such as dust or cats, can provoke an allergy flare-up. Exercise, cold weather, and viral respiratory infections can trigger an asthma attack in many people. Knowing your triggers may help you avoid potentially serious situations. Following are some guidelines to help you anticipate and head off exercise-related allergy and asthma problems before they occur.

Allergic Rhinitis

Most individuals with allergic rhinitis find that certain seasons or environmental surroundings trigger their allergy symptoms. Knowing, for example, that every autumn triggers a hay fever flare-up, you may choose to either avoid exercising outdoors or premedicate with an antihistamine when summer ends. If you have a significant allergy to dust mites and your gym is quite dusty, you again might premedicate before your workout or, in the worst case scenario, change to a cleaner gym. If you have a pollen allergy and the pollen count is high on your outdoor run day, devise a backup plan for indoor exercise that day. Learn to anticipate the potential difficulties your allergies might cause and devise a plan to overcome them and keep your workout schedule on track.

Asthma

Similar to allergic rhinitis, environmental factors, such as dust or pollen, may exacerbate asthma symptoms or trigger an actual asthma attack. As previously discussed, another common trigger for asthma flare-ups is exercise. If you are a person with a known history of exercise-induced asthma, make a plan in advance to prevent symptoms or decrease them once they occur. The most common method of exercise-induced asthma (EIA) prevention is to know your triggers and use your bronchodilator, such as albuterol, before starting your exercise routine that day. Always carry your inhaler and (if needed) delivery device (spacer) with you, either on your person or in your nearby gym bag. If you begin to have shortness of breath or chest tightness, you do not want to be caught without your rescue medication. Knowing your triggers is important if you have antigen-induced asthma. As with allergic rhinitis, if you are going to work out in a facility that has a lot of dust, and dust mites trigger your asthma symptoms, you should either premedicate or choose a different workout

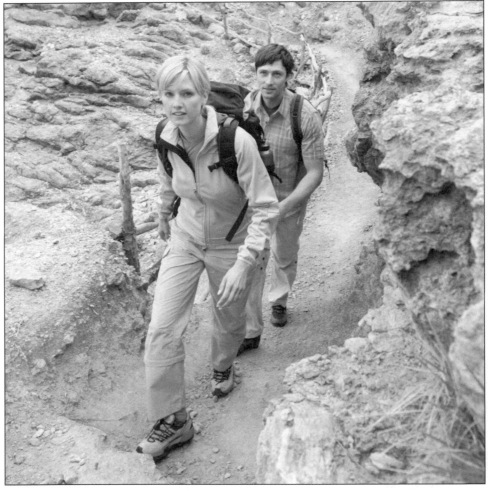

© Jumpfoto

Carrying a bag when possible during exercise is a good way to keep your inhaler and other medications close at hand.

location. If you are going to train outside and you have asthma triggered by pollen or hay fever allergens, check the daily pollen counts with the local weather service. Have an alternate workout plan for those days when your planned training regimen might increase your chance of having an asthma attack. Remember that asthma and allergies should not prevent you from exercising, but you should have a prepared plan of action to prevent and treat flare-ups so that they don't interfere with your workouts.

Expecting the Unexpected

When you are in the middle of your training schedule, certain problems can arise that may derail your best attempts at staying on track with your workouts. Nevertheless, you can still often anticipate and prepare for these surprises. Expect that at some point during your training, disruptions will occur. If you formulate a broad plan for returning to your workouts, you can get back on track easily.

Gym Closures

Fitness clubs have a knack for closing, sometimes unexpectedly. Holidays, renovations, and construction may force your gym to close, a frustrating experience if you do not expect it. However, if you anticipate that at some time you may have to train at a different location, you can easily go with plan B and continue to train. Come up with an alternate routine, perhaps one that you can do at home or one that involves outside exercise. Find another facility nearby for last-minute workouts. Having an alternative option will let you continue working out without skipping a beat.

Illness

Colds and upper respiratory infections can occur at any time of year, although the highest incidence is in the fall and winter months. Most adults average 3 or 4 mild viral respiratory infections each year, but those who spend time with small children tend to get sick more often. Toddlers and preschoolers, especially those in a day care setting, average 8 to 10 viral respiratory infections a year! When your symptoms are mild and you do not have a fever or chest infection, physicians often recommend that you continue to exercise. Mild activity, such as a short walk or stretching, may have a positive benefit on your immune system function, allow you to aerate your lungs better, and help you clear away respiratory secretions. Fever, however, is a sign that you have a more serious illness and your body needs rest. You should not exercise if you have a fever (oral temperature over 101 degrees Fahrenheit); the increased body temperature will predispose you to heat illness and dehydration, both of which can have quite serious ramifications. Drinking plenty of fluids and performing light range of motion exercises are important for maintaining hydration and avoiding stiffness.

Individuals with asthma need to be especially cautious during the cold season. Viral upper respiratory infections are notorious for triggering asthma attacks and wheezing, especially in people with a history of atopic disease (allergic rhinitis, asthma, or eczema). Viral infections, particularly in cold weather, may trigger an asthma attack more easily in someone with a history of EIA because all three factors can decrease the threshold for bronchospasm, or wheezing. As discussed earlier, premedicating with a bronchodilator before exercise may prevent an attack. You will hopefully stop an asthma attack from worsening by also knowing how to recognize your early symptoms of an asthma exacerbation and treating yourself right away with your rescue medication. Always have an asthma action plan (page 7) worked out with your physician ahead of time and know who to call or where to go if your symptoms do not improve quickly.

Injuries

Injuries can derail the best laid exercise plans of even the most motivated and careful exercise aficionado. History tells us that every athlete will likely suffer an injury at some point during his or her training. As discussed previously, strength training is quite safe and, if performed with proper form in a supervised setting, results in few serious injuries. Of course, more vigorous exercise, such as running, jogging, or cycling can incur risks such as overuse and acute traumatic injuries. Overuse injuries, such as stress fractures and tendinitis, can be very debilitating and cause athletes to miss months of training. Similarly, acute injuries, such as an ankle sprain, can require long rehabilitation periods, depending on the severity of the injury.

While not all activity-related injuries can be prevented, common sense and proper equipment go a long way in decreasing the risk. To avoid overtraining, always leave rest days for your body to recuperate. When increasing the intensity of your training, whether the distance run or the amount of weight lifted, be sure to go up slowly. A great rule of thumb is to increase by 5 to 10 percent each week, because increasing the intensity too quickly can lead to conditions such as stress fractures. Always run or jog on well-lit paths, wear reflective clothing at night, and watch the road ahead for holes or uneven surfaces. You should run against the direction of traffic when on roadways shared with automobiles. When cycling, wear a helmet. Protective headgear prevents 80 to 85 percent of severe head trauma and brain damage associated with bicycle accidents. In fact, physicians recommend wearing a helmet any time you are on wheeled devices, such as roller skates, in-line skates, and skateboards. Always have a light on your bike for the dark, wear reflective clothing, and bike in the direction of traffic. Consider having a gait analysis performed by a local therapy center or running group to check for any problems with your biomechanics. Errors in your stride may lead to chronic pain and injury. If you are weight training, have a training partner for spotting on heavier weight sets and always maintain proper technique. If you cannot maintain proper form, the weight is too heavy.

So, if an injury occurs, how do you know whether or not it is serious? Should you treat it yourself or go to see a doctor? While there is no general rule to indicate whether an injury is serious, here are a couple of general guidelines to help you decide if and when you should seek medical attention.

Overuse injuries develop over time and have a gradual onset in pain. Examples of common overuse injuries include tendinitis, bursitis, and chronic muscle strains. Treatment includes rest, either through decreasing activity or changing activity to one that does not cause pain. Ice massage helps decrease inflammation, but remember to avoid frostbite by limiting cold contact to no more than 20 minutes at a time and no more often than every 2 hours. Heat and massage may help decrease stiffness and improve circulation. Pain after exercise that lasts more than a few days should probably be evaluated by a physician. In addition, you should see a doctor if your pain is negatively affecting your workout, causing you to miss days of training, or interfering with your activities of daily living.

In terms of acute injuries, such as ankle sprains or pulled muscles, let pain guide your decision making. In the acute setting you can follow the RICE treatment plan as outlined in the following sidebar to decrease pain and swelling. However, serious symptoms warrant medical attention. If you cannot put pressure or weight on an injured limb, you should see a physician. You should also seek medical attention if you see an obvious deformity or you have pinpoint tenderness over a bone. If you have any pain or movement disturbance (e.g., a limp) that does not resolve within several days, you should see a physician.

Injury Care

Following are the steps in the **RICE** treatment plan for pain relief and swelling:

R = Rest: Decrease activity to a level that does not cause pain. Stop all intense activity until pain diminishes. Continue with light range of motion exercise to avoid joint stiffness.

I = Ice: Ice is an ideal anti-inflammatory agent; however, frostbite can occur. Place a layer of plastic or cloth between the ice and your skin, or constantly move the ice with ice massage. Ice for a maximum of 20 minutes at a time every 2 or 3 hours for the first 48 to 72 hours.

C = Compression: Wrap the joint with a gentle compression wrap, such as an ACE bandage, to decrease fluid accumulation.

E = Elevation: When resting, try to elevate the joint at a level above the heart to decrease swelling.

Some health professionals advocate including **P**rotection and **M**edication to the prescription, creating **PRICEM:**

P = Protection: Protect the injured area with a splint, brace, or sleeve. You can purchase inexpensive versions at most pharmacies and sporting equipment stores.

M = Medication: Over-the-counter anti-inflammatory medications, such as ibuprofen or naproxen, may help decrease pain and inflammation initially.

Exercise After Surgery

Sometimes injuries are more severe than a flare-up of tendinitis or an ankle sprain. Occasionally an injury or medical condition will require surgery, which can be a huge setback to an active person's exercise program.

Rehabilitation may require a few weeks or months, and your workout may need to be put on hold for a short while. Keeping an open mind and a positive attitude go a long way in helping you get back on track with your life again. This means changing up your exercise plan as well, keeping your routine flexible, and getting back in the swing of things as soon as you are physically able.

Depending on the type of surgery you have had, rehabilitation generally starts within 48 hours afterward. In the hospital where I work, even small children have physical therapists to help get them active again as soon as they are medically stable. Maintaining range of motion, flexibility, and baseline strength is vitally important and has positive benefits on both physical and emotional recovery. If you have no complications from your surgery and your physician gives the green light, it is best to get up and moving as soon as possible. You will likely feel exhausted, but getting mobile helps decrease the risk of blood clots, prevents pneumonia and postoperative fever (by preventing atelectasis, or collapse of air sacs in the lung), helps get your bowels moving again, and prevents muscle stiffness and bed sores. Preventing pneumonia is especially important in individuals with asthma and chronic lung disease because air trapping and atelectasis can occur with these conditions and the exposure to viruses and bacteria in the hospital could lead to serious infections.

If your surgery was for a heart or lung condition, get clearance from your heart or lung specialist before starting your exercise program again. If you had brain or major abdominal surgery, you will also need permission and clearance from the surgeon. With most joint or orthopedic procedures, your surgeon will likely want to get you into physical therapy and rehabilitation as soon as possible. It is very important you follow the recommendations of your surgeon and your therapist to avoid reinjury in the postoperative period. After most bone and joint surgeries, therapists will start you off with stretching and gentle range-of-motion exercises the first week, even while you are still in the hospital. After your discharge, you will continue to see out-patient physical therapists who will move on to more weight-loading exercises in the weeks to follow. Rehabilitation is a gradual process; it takes time for scar tissue to stretch and muscle strength to return. It is important not to neglect cardiovascular fitness in the recovery period, so be sure to ask your therapist and surgeon about recommendations on how to stay heart-healthy postoperatively.

Exercise After an Asthma Attack

If you have a severe asthma exacerbation, you may be unable to work out for several days. As discussed earlier, asthma involves tightening of the airways, mucous production, and airway inflammation. Bronchodilators help resolve the spasm of the airways and may decrease the amount of mucus, but the inflammation in the airway walls persists for several days. Oral steroids, such as prednisone, are usually prescribed to reverse this inflammatory process. I would recommend that you give your airways and lungs a rest before restarting your workout, because reversing the airway inflammation requires several days even on steroids. Restarting exercise too soon could trigger more bronchospasm, wheezing, and shortness of breath.

Once you feel your breathing is back to baseline you may gradually return to your workout. You may want to start with flexibility and stretching first, then low-resistance weight training, followed by light cardiovascular exercises. If you are able to tolerate this lighter schedule without any chest tightness, shortness of breath, wheezing, or fatigue, you may resume your regular schedule at your usual intensity. Contact your physician if any asthma symptoms return.

Flexible Programming

As already discussed, the key to staying on track with your training schedule is anticipating potential problems and formulating alternative workout plans. As mentioned earlier, many times you can preplan for even surprise problems. Some breaks to routine that are more concrete in nature, and therefore can be anticipated more easily, are travel and bad weather.

Travel

Whether for work or vacation, taking time away from your usual schedule to travel can interrupt your regular workout routine. Many times, people find it difficult to get back into the rhythm of their workout when coming back from even a short trip. Luckily, this does not have to be the case. Usually when you travel you know your dates, accommodations, and plans in advance and can easily create alternative workout plans. You have several options depending on where you are going, the local climate, and your accommodation facilities. You can easily use the Internet to investigate your destination ahead of time.

Use the following checklist when researching hotels in advance or planning an alternative workout routine:

- Do accommodations have on-site exercise facilities? Is the price included, or do I have to pay an extra cost?
- What type of equipment is in the facility?
- What are the facility's hours of operation?
- Does a nearby health club or fitness facility offer day passes or short-term access? Does the hotel have a discount agreement with the facility? What is the distance to the facility from the hotel?
- Does the hotel offer any workout suites? (Some hotels now offer special room packages that include a treadmill, yoga mat, and healthy foods in the room for a special price.)

- Is it safe to run, jog, or walk outside in the neighborhood? Are any trails or routes in the vicinity? How long are the trails, and what is the terrain?
- Does the hotel have a pool? Is it indoor or outdoor?
- Can I rent a bicycle for daily use? Are any trails or bike routes in the vicinity? Are helmets available?

When you have reviewed the checklist and know what to anticipate in terms of workout options, develop a tentative training schedule for the time you will spend there. Having a definite plan will allow you to stay on track and avoid procrastination. If you are spending a week at a destination, write down your routine for three of the days and plan to rest on your days off. For example, do upper body weight training at the hotel gym on Monday, walk an hour on Wednesday, and perform lower body strength training on Friday. Walking or jogging is the easiest way to get exercise, especially cardiovascular exercise, into your routine. You need no equipment except a good pair of sturdy shoes, and you can walk just about anywhere. Make sure you check into the safety of the area around the hotel and the availability of any paths or routes. Walking, jogging, or biking around the hotel helps you get to know your new surroundings. Some hotels now offer pedometers that guests can check out to measure the distance. An alternative is to carry a watch and base your exercise on duration. If the local neighborhood is not that safe or the weather is wet, consider walking at a nearby shopping mall or changing to an indoor workout plan.

If you have allergies, check local pollen and mold counts before your trip. Many national weather media outlets offer this information daily, especially during peak allergy season. If allergen counts are high, you may need to bring along antihistamines or choose to exercise indoors. Also, become familiar with your destination's local climate and plan accordingly. When I was at a recent conference in the San Francisco Bay Area, several colleagues who expected warm weather were surprised upon awakening for their early morning run that the air was crisp and cool. Fortunately my friend with asthma had his rescue inhaler with him and avoided a severe acute asthma attack. Some locales are dry and dusty, others are cold and wet, and some have high levels of air pollution and smog. Any one of these factors may trigger allergy symptoms or wheezing in susceptible people and would require vigilance and medication or avoidance to prevent a potentially serious outcome.

Exercising indoors at a hotel is often an easy option. If your destination has a well-equipped fitness facility, you will have no problem continuing your regular workout schedule of weight training, cardiovascular exercise, or both. If the hotel gym is lacking equipment or space, you will have to look at more creative alternatives. Check into local health clubs to see whether they offer day passes or even short-term memberships if you are staying for an extended period. Many times hotels have agreements with local clubs to offer guests discounts or free passes. If you belong to a large national health club chain, see whether they have a facility near your hotel. In the event your hotel is located near a local college or university, you could check into using the fitness facilities on campus (check school holiday schedules!). Another possibility is using a local community center such as a park district gym or a club such as the YMCA. Many times these locales offer visitors temporary access or, as is the case with the YMCA, if you are a member at one branch you can usually use other branches across the country for free.

As a last resort you can always perform a modified workout in your room. Your goal is to maintain some strength and flexibility so that you do not lose your previous gains while you are away. You can easily achieve this goal by using body weight or rubber tubing exercises in your room as well as performing small-scale cardiovascular exercises. You can perform many strength training exercises using your own body weight as resistance. Good basic exercises include abdominal crunches, push-ups, back stabilizing exercises, and wall slides. These exercises can be done daily and provide a great workout for your core muscle groups. Rubber tubing is lightweight, ideal for travel, and fits into any nook or cranny of your luggage. Almost every exercise mentioned in chapter 4 can be performed using rubber tubing as resistance. You can do arm curls (both biceps and triceps) as well as shoulder presses and leg flexion and extension exercises in a hotel room in a short time. Remember to focus on a higher number of low-resistance repetitions to improve endurance, maintaining strict form and proper technique. For cardiovascular exercise, you can easily march or jog in place or perform jumping jacks to work up a sweat and raise your heart rate. The one potential drawback to exercising in your hotel room is dust. Most hotel rooms are carpeted. Dust mites can be lurking under the bed, the desk, and even in the vacuumed main traffic areas. If you have a dust allergy and plan to do exercises on the floor in your room, consider premedicating with an antihistamine to avoid a miserable experience!

Perhaps the most important area of concern when a person with allergies or asthma books a hotel room is whether the room is smoking or not. Smoke residue from cigarettes, pipes, and cigars lingers in carpet, furniture, bedding, and drapes. Even if no one has smoked in a particular room recently, the odor from previous smokers remains. Individuals with even slight smoke allergies may begin experiencing rhinitis symptoms or wheezing within minutes of entering a "smoking" room. For those readers with significant reactions to smoke, you will want to be sure to request nonsmoking rooms when you book a hotel room.

Flexibility is also an important component of the fitness triangle; do not ignore it while traveling. In some ways, a stretching routine is easier to maintain when not at home because you can stretch anywhere. Try to include flexibility training in your daily routine or at least incorporate stretching on the days you perform your strength training or cardiovascular exercises. Some people prefer to stretch in the morning to get the blood flowing and provide for some gentle awakening movements before starting the workday. Others prefer to stretch in the evening, to relax from a busy day and prepare their bodies for sleep. Whichever you choose (or if do both,) be sure to make your stretches as functional and dynamic as possible. Controlled, relaxed breathing and, if possible, a quiet atmosphere are other key components to a beneficial stretching routine.

If your travel involves long car or plane rides, stretching and maintaining flexibility are of paramount importance in staying healthy and free of pain. Prolonged periods of sitting not only lead to joint stiffness but can have serious effects on your general health as well. Individuals who spend many hours seated with their hips and knees flexed are at higher risk for venous stasis (pooling of the blood in the lower extremities) and blood clots. The risk for blood clots may be increased if a person is overweight or has a history of poor circulation, such as sickle cell disease or diabetes, and the risk is also increased at higher altitudes. If you are on a long flight, try to stand up, stretch, and walk around every hour or so to get your muscles moving. Even while seated, try to fully extend your

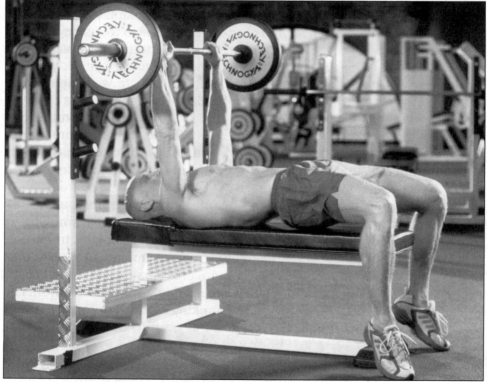

Plan to fit in exercise when you're traveling. Many hotels offer on-site fitness facilities.

knees and hold the stretch several seconds, curl and uncurl your toes, and raise and lower your heels multiple times, repeating often during the flight. Be sure to drink a lot of water and avoid caffeine and alcohol, both of which can be dehydrating.

The key when traveling is to create an alternative workout schedule that is flexible enough to deal with the minor inconveniences of being away from home. Before you leave, investigate possible facilities for strength and cardiovascular training. Consider bringing along lightweight and portable equipment, such as tubing or an exercise mat, to help perform a modified routine in your hotel room. Try to incorporate some type of physical exercise or stretching into your daily schedule every day to keep yourself active and allow you to easily return to your regular workout schedule when you return.

Weather

As we all know, weather can interfere with just about everything, from a walk to the store to a wedding! Rain, snow, sleet, hail, storms, excessive cold, and excessive heat can prevent you from exercising outdoors or simply traveling to the gym. Inclement weather can be tricky to anticipate but, if you resign yourself to the fact that rainy days and snowy days will occur, then you can easily keep your training schedule on track. Choose an alternative place to exercise that is indoor or climate controlled such as a shopping mall or a nearby health club. Perhaps for this type of situation you may want to purchase ahead of time a device that elevates the back wheel of your outdoor bicycle and turns it into an indoor stationary bike. If you live in a cold climate and prefer not to join a health club for the winter months, consider purchasing an indoor stationary bike, elliptical trainer, cross-country ski machine, or treadmill.

Allergy sufferers need to pay special attention to the local environment and weather changes. Exercisers who are sensitive to flowers, trees, grasses, and molds need to check daily pollen and mold counts before exercising outdoors. If you do decide to exercise outside on a day with moderately high pollen counts, be sure to take an antihistamine at least 30 minutes before beginning your routine. In addition, discuss with your physician whether you need a daily nasal steroid during the high risk times of the year, such as hay fever season, to better control your symptoms. If you have moderate to severe asthma that is triggered by environmental allergens, such as pollen, be sure to have your rescue inhaler on hand during your run or jog. In fact, you should probably take two puffs of the inhaler approximately 10 to 15 minutes before exercising to prevent the onset of asthma symptoms. Premedication with albuterol is especially important during cold weather, which may provoke an asthma attack in many exercisers with asthma. The bottom line in avoiding significant allergy or asthma symptoms with outdoor exercise is, know the current weather outside before opening the door.

In case of inclement or allergy-provoking weather, your backup plan could be as simple as performing strength and flexibility exercises at home using your body weight, handheld weights, or rubber tubing. Invest a small amount of money to keep a stash of basic equipment such as an exercise mat, rubber tubing, and a few sizes of handheld dumbbells. This way you always have a low-cost, last-minute exercise option on hand. As with the travel program, basic exercises to include are those that focus on core strength muscle groups such as abdominals, chest, pelvic stabilizers, and back as well as thigh muscles. If the forecast is for storms all week, plan out a few days' worth of exercises, perhaps grouping chest and triceps one day, back and biceps another day, and back and abdominal exercises on the third day. Crunches, push-ups, bird-dog, plinth, and wall slides need no special equipment. You can do arm curls, shoulder presses, and leg strengthening exercises with rubber tubing. You can still do your usual flexibility program, which is usually performed indoors. Making a backup plan that you can easily substitute for your planned workout on days with bad weather lets you maintain your strength and flexibility until you are able to return to the gym.

Hot Weather

Exercising in high heat can be quite dangerous. Most people are well aware of the dangers of heatstroke because of recent high-profile deaths of college and professional athletes. Heat illness encompasses a variety of conditions, from mild heat cramps to severe heat exhaustion to life-threatening heatstroke. Heat illness occurs when the body's capacity to store heat outpaces its ability to lose heat; in other words, heat generated by working muscles overcomes the sweating and heat loss mechanisms of the body. The frequency of heat illness depends on the air temperature, humidity, and thus the heat index. Risk factors for heat illness include obesity, dehydration, fatigue, prior history of heat illness, fever, imperme-able clothing, and certain supplements and medications. Symptoms of heatstroke include headache, dizziness, fatigue, irritability, anxiety, chills, nausea, vomiting, and severe cramps. More serious symptoms include confusion and change in mental status, seizures, and loss of consciousness. Elevated core body temperature and a cessation of sweating are ominous signs of heatstroke, the fatality rate of which is quite high.

ACSM has developed guidelines for preventing heat illness (2005). These guidelines include:

1. Plan outdoor activities based on the heat index. Avoid strenuous exercise when the air temperature is above 90 degrees Fahrenheit and the humidity is over 65 percent. See the heat index scale in figure 8.1.
2. Exercise early in the morning or late in the evening to avoid the hottest times of the day.

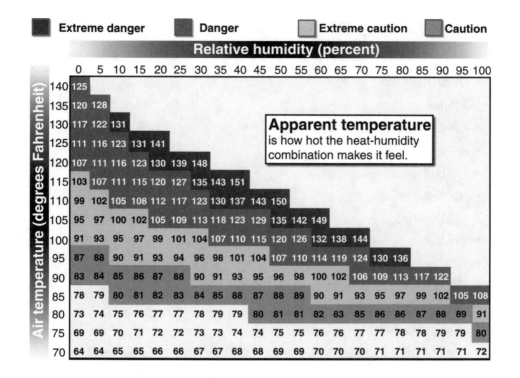

Figure 8.1 Heat index scale.
From National Oceanographic and Atmospheric Administration.

3. Acclimate yourself to the temperature. If you are moving from Maine to Phoenix, try to allow at least 10 days for your body and, more importantly, your body's heat loss mechanisms to progressively adjust to the new climate before exercising strenuously outdoors.

4. Use physical barriers for protection from sun and heat, such as light-colored, lightweight clothing and a hat or visor.

5. Stop taking medications that impair heat loss (see following text).

6. Prehydrate your body, and drink often during exercise. (See the following text for determining how much to drink based on sweat rate.)

7. Move exercise to shady, cool areas or indoors on very hot days.

8. Decrease the intensity of your outdoor workout, and monitor yourself for signs of heat illness.

The exact risk of dehydration depends on the individual's heat loss mechanisms, primarily the sweat rate. Calculating the sweat rate is not as complicated as it sounds and is actually a good idea for anyone who likes to exercise outdoors. You can calculate you own sweat rate by weighing yourself without clothes before exercise and again after exercise. Subtract the weights (in pounds), and account for any fluid (in ounces) you drank

Symptoms and Signs of Heat Illness

▶ Headache

▶ Dizziness

▶ Fatigue

▶ Irritability

▶ Anxiety

▶ Chills and profuse sweating

▶ Nausea or vomiting

▶ Heat cramps

▶ Confusion or mental status changes*

▶ Seizures*

▶ Rapid breathing or rapid heart rate*

▶ Low blood pressure*

▶ Elevated body temperature*

▶ Loss of consciousness*

▶ Core temperature over 106 degrees Fahrenheit and cessation of sweating*

    * = ominous sign of life-threatening heatstroke

From the ACSM Position Stand: *Heat and Cold Illnesses and Long Distance Runners,* 1996, and ACSM's Inter-Association Task Force on Exertional Heat Illnesses Consensus Statement.

during exercise. The answer is the amount of sweat you lost from that exercise. Now correct for the amount of time: You want your sweat rate per hour, so if you exercised for an hour and a half you have to divide the number by 1.5. So, to replenish this lost fluid you must drink 2 cups of fluid (16 ounces) for every pound of body weight lost. Divide this amount so that you are drinking fluids every 15 to 20 minutes during exercise, 10 to 20 ounces 2 hours before exercise, and 20 to 30 ounces after exercise.

Certain medications and supplements can increase the risk of heat illness and dehydration. This factor is especially important for people with allergic diseases who take antihistamines and decongestants to control their symptoms. Antihistamines can be detrimental in two ways: they can impair the body's ability to dissipate (lose) heat and their side effects may mimic the symptoms of serious heat illnesses. Antihistamines, both first and second generation, can impair heat loss and increase the risk of heat illness. In addition, common side effects of antihistamines include dry ("cotton") mouth, decreased urinary output, and confusion. These effects could mask symptoms of heat exhaustion or heatstroke and might delay someone from seeking potentially life-saving medical attention.

Nasal decongestants may have a diuretic effect on the kidneys, increasing water loss and thus the risk for dehydration. Most sports physicians would advise stopping antihistamines and decongestants before strenuous exercise in hot environs. Another alternative is to change the patient to a nasal steroid for localized control of allergic-associated congestion and runny nose without the generalized effects on heat loss.

Cold Weather

Just like strenuous exercise in the heat, exercising in the cold requires knowing the risks and taking certain precautions. The primary health risks associated with exercising in cold weather include hypothermia and frostbite, although cold-related allergic diseases occur as well.

Most people assume they can only get hypothermia if it is freezing cold outside with blowing snow and frigid winds. However, hypothermia can happen all too often on cool, sunny autumn or spring days as well as in the dead of winter. You can even get hypothermia exercising in wet clothes after a summer thunderstorm! Unfortunately, I have had personal experience covering events such as the Chicago Marathon where, on a crisp and sunny fall day we sent several people to the emergency room for cold-related illness. The important fact to remember is that cold illnesses can usually be prevented through simple precautions.

Hypothermia occurs when the body's core temperature drops below 95 degrees Fahrenheit. Risk factors include the extremes of age (under 18 and over 65), dehydration, malnutrition, certain medical illnesses, and some medications. Exposure to the cold results in peripheral vasoconstriction, and the blood vessels of the hands and feet clamp down to shunt warm blood to the vital organs. This unfortunately predisposes the extremities more to tissue damage from prolonged exposure. Also in individuals who are strenuously exercising and are already losing heat rapidly from their active muscles, the cold air will exacerbate the heat loss. The cold also directly affects the central nervous system, depressing activity and producing symptoms of confusion, slurred speech, emotional lability (laughing then crying), and impaired memory. Breathing may be initially fast and then slow as brain function slows. Heart rhythm disturbances, erratic breathing, and a fall in blood pressure can lead to loss of consciousness and even death. Rapid rewarming and medical attention are the keys to successful treatment.

Frostbite is tissue damage from exposure to the cold. The longer an extremity is exposed to cold air or cold water, the more damage that is likely to occur. Body parts with the highest risks of frostbite include feet and hands, ears, nose, and the cheeks. Symptoms include numbness, tingling, pain, and clumsiness. Blisters can form as well, but pain usually does not occur until the area is warmed. Superficial frostbite has normal skin color, normal sensation, skin that indents with gentle pressure, and blisters with clear fluid. Deep frostbite has bluish-white skin that does not indent upon touching and remains numb, as well as small blood-filled blisters. Superficial frostbite has a better prognosis than deep frostbite. Rewarming and then freezing again can result in worse tissue damage, so rewarming should not be started until refreezing can be prevented. Skin that is exposed to the cold and upon rewarming has normal color, normal sensation, and no blisters will likely be fine. Any skin that has abnormal color, remains numb after rewarming, or has blisters should be seen by a physician.

ACSM has developed guidelines for avoiding exposure to extreme temperatures for distance runners. The recommendations for preventing hypothermia and frostbite include the following:

1. Ensure good conditioning and proper baseline nutrition.
2. Acclimate to the cold environment slowly over several days.
3. Avoid alcohol and smoking.
4. Dress in layers. The layer closest to the skin should be a synthetic material that wicks away moisture from the skin, the middle layer is optional but should be one that traps heat well, and the outer layer should be waterproof or water resistant.
5. Wear lightweight, windproof materials and keep them loose to trap a cushion of dry, warm air above the skin.
6. Cover your head; it is a major source of heat loss.
7. Wear a scarf or face mask in extremely cold weather or if you have cold-induced allergic disease (see following text).
8. Wear mittens if you can; they keep the fingers together, thereby reducing heat loss.
9. If you are exercising in a temperature below freezing (less than 32 degrees Fahrenheit), choose three layers as described previously for hands and feet.

From the ACSM Position Stand: *Heat and Cold Illnesses and Long Distance Runners,* 1996, and ACSM's Inter-Association Task Force on Exertional Heat Illnesses Consensus Statement.

Individuals with certain allergic diseases, such as cold urticaria and asthma, need to maintain special caution in cold weather. A relatively small group of people get urticaria or hives when their skin is exposed to cold air or water. They need to have all skin as covered as possible and wear water-resistant outer layers. If their reaction is severe they might need to avoid being out in cold weather at all. Exposure to cold air is a common trigger for asthma attacks among people with EIA as well as asthma. Breathing in cold, dry air can directly trigger bronchospasm, or tightening of the airway, leading to wheezing, coughing, shortness of breath, and chest pain. A small group of people with asthma rarely get asthma symptoms under normal ambient conditions, but when exercising in cold weather get asthma attacks. Covering the nose and mouth with a scarf or face mask will allow the air to warm briefly before entering the airway, thereby reducing the likelihood of bronchospasm. If you have airways that are extremely sensitive to cold air, you may need to pre-medicate with albuterol or another bronchodilator before going outside to exercise in cold weather. All people with asthma would be wise to have their bronchodilator inhaler on their person while exercising, especially in cold weather, in case they develop respiratory symptoms.

Anticipating the possibility of weather-related problems and taking steps to prevent them are important for all outdoor athletes. The extremes of temperature can lead to sometimes serious medical conditions and may trigger allergic conditions in certain individuals. Knowing how to prevent such injuries through proper attire, timing of exercise, and possible medication use, or avoidance, is critical. Being able to recognize the early signs and symptoms of temperature-related injuries may facilitate early and therefore more successful treatment.

Avoiding Boredom

Perhaps one of the biggest detractors from staying on track with an exercise plan is the "I don't feel like it" phenomenon. We have all had days when we do not feel we have the energy or desire to go to the gym and work out. This feeling is human nature and, if it is short lived, may not be such a bad thing. Perhaps it is your body's way of saying you need a day off to rest and recuperate. Perhaps it is your mind's way of telling you to dedicate the day to other items on your "to do" list to avoid procrastination stress later on. The real question is, Why do you feel that way? Is it a once-in-a-while occurrence, or is the feeling of skipping a workout becoming more and more frequent? Are you tired or depressed in general? Are you stressed from some other aspect of life, or are you just bored with your workout?

If you truly feel depressed or fatigued, you should not ignore these symptoms. Fatigue, extreme tiredness, or boredom with many aspects of life may be a manifestation of a serious medical condition. Fatigue can be a sign of a depleted immune system and could predispose you to recurrent infections. Low energy levels could represent anemia, especially in menstruating females or individuals with poor nutrition. Hypothyroidism, depression, and bipolar disorder are all treatable conditions that present with fatigue. Even if you are tired because of stress or too much work, unusual fatigue is a warning sign that something is wrong and needs to be investigated.

Often when people do not want to train it is because they have become bored with their routine. As with any other activity, going through the same motions day after day can become monotonous and tedious.

So, people often ask me, "How can I keep my routine fresh?" You can do several things to shake up your routine. First, you can alter your program by changing the exercises to make it more interesting. If you always do bench press with dumbbells on a flat bench for chest, change it up and try a chest press on an incline or decline bench, or try cable crossover flys. You can also change the resistance or number of sets and repetitions. For example, if you usually do 3 sets of 12 repetitions for each exercise, you could change to 4 sets of increasing resistance and decreasing number of repetitions (e.g., first set 12 reps at 50 percent maximum weight, next set 10 reps at 60 percent maximum weight, next set 8 reps at 65 percent maximum weight, and last set 6 reps at 70 percent maximum). Keep your new routine for 4 to 6 weeks, then make some changes again.

You can also alter your balance of strength training, cardiovascular exercise, and stretching to add a little kick to your routine. For example, if you normally weight train 3 days a week and run 2 days a week, mix it up and change to weight training 2 days a week, swimming 2 days a week, and 1 day of flexibility exercises. Stick to your new schedule for several weeks, then make another alteration to keep it fresh. Perhaps the best way to jump-start your routine is to find a workout partner. As mentioned before, exercising with another person can give a big boost to your workout and motivate you to work harder and thus increase your gains.

When you start to train, you get into a good rhythm. Your training is producing endorphins, and you feel good about yourself. You look better, feel stronger, and have a more positive outlook. As you achieve a higher level of cardiovascular fitness you may also see your asthma come under better control. You also see the progress you are making in the gym, which motivates you to stick with your program. When I really get into my routine, I feel down the days I cannot make it to the gym for a workout because of work or other projects. However, if I stop working out for an extended time, I often find it is very difficult to get back into the swing of my routine. Sometimes it is hard to muster the energy to get back to the gym to start training again. That is why this chapter is so important. These feelings are natural and normal but still detrimental to our overall plan of living a healthy lifestyle. We all need to come up with backup plans to help us get back to our training routine. This is where having a written alternative workout or a training partner are especially useful. The idea is to find something unique to you that will help motivate you to get back on track with your training schedule.

Summary

Sticking with an exercise program is often challenging. Many pitfalls and obstacles interfere with our ability to stick with our planned routine. Dealing with allergies, asthma, and other allergic diseases is another potential barrier to staying on track. You now know several ways of avoiding pitfalls, anticipating possible setbacks, and preemptively dealing with those problems to stick with the program. Keys to staying on track with exercise include setting and reviewing your exercise goals, organizing a fun and flexible routine, and preparing for potential pitfalls.

Asthma and allergies should not prevent you from exercising and staying fit. In fact, the exact opposite is true. The benefits your body, especially your cardiovascular system, receives from regular exercise will help you live a long and healthy life. Allergic disease and asthma are small road bumps that you need to address but can easily overcome. Taking logical steps to avoid potential triggers, taking your medication correctly, and learning to recognize the early symptoms of serious allergic conditions are the keys you need to exercise successfully. This book provides you with some useful tips to design a new exercise program or improve your current one, whether you have mild allergic rhinitis or severe allergic disease. In the end our goal is the same: stay healthy; stay strong; and live a long, happy life.

ACTION PLAN:

STAYING ON TRACK TO REDUCE SYMPTOMS

☐ Set both short-term and long-term goals that are realistic and attainable.

☐ Develop a simple, fun routine to meet your goals.

☐ Write down your exercise plan. Keep a log book or calendar so that you know what you should be doing on a specific day.

☐ Review your goals regularly and alter your routine to keep meeting your objectives.

☐ Be flexible in your approach to exercise. Be willing to adapt your routine to adjust to future potential obstacles or flare-ups of your allergic disease.

☐ Anticipate potential problem areas and develop a contingency plan ahead of time so that when the problem presents itself you don't get sidetracked or fall behind in your training.

☐ Develop plans to continue exercising during travel, adverse weather, and potential allergy-triggering conditions.

☐ Have a good support system. A training partner is ideal.

☐ Keep your routine interesting and fresh by making frequent alterations so that you enjoy your program and avoid plateaus.

☐ Have fun!

REFERENCES

American College of Sports Medicine (ACSM). 2005. *ACSM's guidelines for exercise testing and prescription.* 7th ed. Baltimore: Lippincott Williams & Wilkins.

Armstrong, L.E., Y. Epstein, J.E. Greenleaf, E.M. Haymes, R.W. Hubbard, W.O. Roberts, and P.D. Thompson. 1996. American College of Sports Medicine position stand: Heat and cold illnesses during distance running. *Medicine & Science in Sports & Exercise* 28(12):i-x.

Bera, T.K., and M.V. Rajapurkar. 1993. Body composition, cardiovascular endurance, and aerobic power of yoga practitioners. *Indian Journal of Physiology and Pharmacology* 37:225-228.

Bock, S.A. 1987. Prospective appraisal of complaints of adverse reactions to foods in children in the first 3 years of life. *Pediatrics* 79(5):683-688.

Clark, C.J. 1993. The role of physical training in asthma. *In Principles and practice of pulmonary rehabilitation,* R. Casaburi and T.L. Petty, 424-438. Philadelphia: W.B. Saunders.

Faigenbaum, A.D. 2000. Strength training for children and adolescents. *Clinics in Sports Medicine* 19(4, October):593-619.

Fitch, K.D., A.R. Morton, and B.A. Blanksby. 1976. Effects of swimming training on children with asthma. *Archives of Childhood Diseases* 51:190-194.

Hickson, R.C., C. Foster, M.L. Pollock, and S. Rich. 1985. Reduced training intensities and loss of aerobic power, endurance, and cardiac growth. *Journal of Applied Physiology* 58:492-499.

Huovinen, E., J. Kaprio, and L.A. Laitinen. 2001. Social predictor of adult asthma: A co-twin case-control study. *Thorax* 56:234-236.

Joshi, L.N., V.D. Joshi, and L.V. Gokhale. 1992. Effect of short term 'Pranayam' practice on breathing rate and ventilatory functions of lung. *Indian Journal of Physiology and Pharmacology* 36:105-108.

Knowler, W.C., E. Barret-Conner, S.E. Fowler, et al. 2002. Reduction in the incidence of type 2 diabetes with lifestyle intervention or metformin. *New England Journal of Medicine* 346(6):393-403.

Kohrt, W.M., S.A. Bloomfield, K.D. Little, M.E. Nelson, and V.R. Yingling. 2004. American College of Sports Medicine position stand: Physical activity and bone health. *Medicine & Science in Sports & Exercise* 36(11):1986-1996.

Krause W.E., J.A. Houmard, B.D. Duscha, et al. 2002. Effects of the amount and intensity of exercise on plasma lipoproteins. *New England Journal of Medicine* 347:1483-1492.

Lloyd, L.K. 2001. Are you ready to exercise? How to start an exercise program. *The Fit Society Page* (Summer):1,5.

Makwana, K., N. Khirwadkar, and H.C. Gupta. 1988. Effect of short-term yoga practice on ventilatory function tests. *Indian Journal of Physiology and Pharmacology* 32:202-208.

McKenzie, D.C., S.L. McLuckie, and D.R. Stirling. 1994. The protective effects of continuous and interval exercise in athletes with exercise induced asthma. *Medicine & Science in Sports & Exercise* 26:951-956.

Minor, M.A., J.E. Hewett, R.R. Webel, S.K. Anderson, and D.R. Kay. 1989. Efficacy of physical conditioning in patients with rheumatoid arthritis and osteoarthritis. *Arthritis and Rheumatism* 32(11):1396-1405.

Orenstein, D.M. 2002. Pulmonary problems and management in youth sports. *Pediatric Clinics of North America* 49:709-721.

Pollock, M.L., G.A. Gaesser, J.D. Butcher, J. Despres, R.K. Dishman, B.A. Franklin, and C.E. Garber. 1998. ACSM position stand: The recommended quantity and quality of exercise for developing and maintaining cardiorespiratory and muscular fitness, and flexibility in healthy adults. *Medicine & Science in Sports & Exercise* 30(6):975-991.

Prochaska, J.O., and C.C. DiClemente. 1983. Stages and processes of self-change of smoking: Toward an integrative model of change. *Journal of Consulting and Clinical Psychology* 51:390-395.

Rai, L., and K. Ram. 1993. Energy expenditure and ventilatory response during Virasana— a yogic standing posture. *Indian Journal of Physiology and Pharmacology* 37:45-50.

Raju, P.S., K.V. Prasad, R.Y. Venkata, K.J. Murthy, and M.V. Reddy. 1997. Influences of intensive yoga training on physiologic changes in 6 adult women: A case report. *Journal of Alternative and Complimentary Medicine* 3:291-295.

Rasmussen, F., J. Lambrechtsen, H.C. Siersted, H.S. Hansen, and H.C. Hansen. 2000. Low physical fitness in childhood is associated with the development of asthma in young adulthood: The Odense schoolchild study. *European Respiratory Journal* 16:866-870.

Ray, U.S., S. Mukhopadhaya, S.S. Purkayastha, V. Ansani, O.S. Tomer, R. Prashad, L. Thakur, and W. Selvmurthy. 2001. Effect of yogic exercises on physical and mental health of young fellowship course trainees. *Indian Journal of Physiology and Pharmacology* 45:37-53.

Reiff, D.B., N.B. Choudry, N.B. Pride, and P.W. Ind. 1989. The effect of prolonged submaximal warm-up exercise on exercise induced asthma. *American Review of Respiratory Disease* 139(2):479-484.

Robertson, R.J., F.L. Goss, J. Dube, J. Rutkowski, M. Dupain, C. Brennan, and J. Andreacci. 2004. Validation of the adult OMNI scale of perceived exertion for cycle ergometer exercise. *Medicine & Science in Sports & Exercise* 36(1):102-108.

Sabina, A.B., A.L. Williams, H.K. Wall, S. Bansal, G. Chupp, and D.L. Kats. 2005. Yoga intervention for adults with mild-to-moderate asthma: A pilot study. *Annals of Allergy, Asthma, and Immunology* 95(4):543-548.

Satta, A. 2000. Exercise training in asthma. *Journal of Sports Medicine and Physical Fitness* 40:277-283.

Telles S., S.K. Reddy, and H.R. Nagendra. 2000. Oxygen consumption and respiration following two yoga relaxation techniques. *Applied Psychophysiology Feedback* 25:221-227.

Tran, M.D., R.G. Holly, J. Lashbrook, and E.A. Amsterdam. 2001. Effects of hatha yoga practice on health related aspects of physical fitness. *Preventive Cardiology* 4:165-170.

U.S. Department of Health and Human Services. 1996. Physical activity and health: A report of the Surgeon General. Centers for Disease Control and Prevention, National Center for Chronic Disease Prevention and Health Promotion. www.cdc.gov (accessed April 26, 2006.)

Vickers, A.J., and C. Smith. 1997. Analysis of the evidence profile of the effectiveness of complimentary therapies in asthma: A qualitative survey and systematic review. *Complementary Therapies in Medicine* 5(4):202-209.

Weber, R.W. Meteorologic variables in aerobiology. *Immunology and Allergy Clinics of North America* 23:411-422 (table 1).

Wei, M., L.W. Gibbons, T.L. Mitchell, J.B. Kampert, C.D. Lee, and S.N. Blair. 1999. The association between cardiorespiratory fitness and impaired fasting glucose and type 2 diabetes mellitus in men. *Annals of Internal Medicine* 130:89-96.

Wolf, S.L., H.X. Barnhart, G.L. Ellison, and C.E. Coogler. 1997. The effects of Tai Chi Quan and computerized balance training on postural stability in older adults. Atlanta FICSIT Group: Frailty and injuries: Cooperative studies on intervention techniques. *Physical Therapy* 77(4):371-381.

INDEX

Note: The italicized *f* and *t* refer to figures and tables, respectively.

ABOUT THE AUTHOR

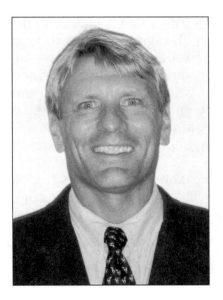

Dr. William Briner is the medical director for the Sports Medicine Center and director of the Primary Care Sports Medicine Fellowship at Lutheran General Hospital in Park Ridge, Illinois. He was the physician for the indoor volleyball venue during the 1996 and 2004 Olympic Games and has served as the team physician for the U.S. national soccer and volleyball teams as well as for local high school and college teams. Dr. Briner's research interests include preparticipation examinations for sports, ankle sprains, volleyball injuries, and allergic conditions related to exercise. Dr. Briner is a fellow of the American College of Sports Medicine.

ABOUT THE CONTRIBUTORS

Jeffrey M. Mjaanes, MD, has been a practicing assistant professor of pediatrics at Rush University Medical Center in Chicago since 2002. In June 2006 he will complete a sports medicine fellowship position at Advocate Lutheran General Hospital in Park Ridge, Illinois. Dr. Mjaanes graduated from the University of Wisconsin at Madison, where he was a Spanish and international relations major. He went on to complete medical school at the University of Wisconsin and his pediatric residency at Rush. Dr. Mjaanes and his wife, Mercedes, have two daughters, Gabriela and Lucia.

Matthew J. Brandon, MD, is currently medical director of Family Health and Fitness Specialists, Ltd., in South Elgin, Illinois. In June 2006 he completed a sports medicine fellowship through Advocate Lutheran General Hospital in Park Ridge, Illinois. Dr. Brandon completed his family medicine residency at MacNeal Hospital in Berwyn, Illinois, and medical school at the University of Illinois College of Medicine. He is interested in endurance sports, exercise physiology, and injury prevention. Dr. Brandon and his wife, Charlotte, have one son, Nathan, and enjoy travel and downhill skiing.

ABOUT ACSM

The American College of Sports Medicine (ACSM) is more than the world's leader in the fields of sports medicine and exercise science—it is an association of people and professions exploring the use of that science and physical activity to make life healthier for all people.

Since 1954, ACSM has been committed to the promotion of physical activity and the diagnosis, treatment, and prevention of sport-related injuries. With more than 20,000 international, national, and regional chapter members in 80 countries, ACSM is internationally known as the leading source of state-of-the-art research and information on sports medicine and exercise science. Through ACSM, health and fitness professionals representing a variety of disciplines work to improve the quality of life for people around the world through health and fitness research, education, and advocacy.

A large part of ACSM's mission is devoted to public awareness and education about the positive aspects of physical activity for people of all ages from all walks of life. ACSM's physicians, researchers, and educators have created tools for the public, ranging in scope from starting an exercise program to avoiding or treating sport injuries.

ACSM's National Center is located in Indianapolis, Indiana, widely recognized as the amateur sports capitol of the nation. To learn more about ACSM, visit www.acsm.org.

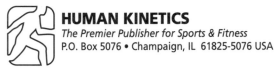